NATUROPATHIC MEDI

Explains the principles on which naturopathy is based and outlines the naturopathic procedures which are used diagnostically and therapeutically in modern practice.

By the same author:
DIETS TO HELP CONTROL CHOLESTEROL
DIETS TO HELP HAY FEVER AND ASTHMA
DIETS TO HELP HEART DISORDERS
FIRST-AID — NATURE'S WAY
PRINCIPLES AND PRACTICE OF MOXIBUSTION
(co-authored with Royston Low)
SELF-HELP FOR GALL BLADDER TROUBLES

NATUROPATHIC MEDICINE

Treating the Whole Person

by

Roger Newman Turner
N.D., D.O., B.Ac., M.B.N.O.A.

Series Editor

Dr George T. Lewith

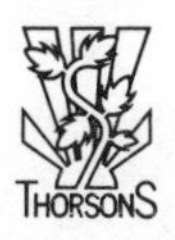

THORSONS PUBLISHERS LIMITED
Wellingborough, Northamptonshire

First published 1984
Second Impression February 1985
Third Impression June 1985

British Library Cataloguing in Publication Data

Newman Turner, R.
Naturopathic medicine.
1. Naturopathy
I. Title
615.5'35 RZ440

ISBN 0-7225-0785-2

Printed and Bound in Great Britain by
Whitstable Litho Ltd., Whitstable, Kent

For Birgid,
Nicole and Julian

Acknowledgements

It takes many different views to mould a profession and, to fairly describe one as wide-ranging as naturopathy, it was necessary that I should speak with practitioners of various persuasions rather than rely solely on my own experience. I am grateful to the many colleagues around the world with whom I have discussed naturopathic medicine, but in particular to Albert Priest, Keki Sidhwa, Erich Weiss, and Brian K. Youngs, who gave generously of their time to consider the basic principles and various aspects of its practice.

The helpful comments and criticisms made by Dr George Lewith, the series editor, and John Hardaker, Editorial Director of Thorsons Publishers, are also much appreciated. Birgid Newman Turner has patiently guided me through a number of German textbooks and technical papers.

My greatest appreciation, however, must be expressed to Lynne Gerrard, who, amidst her many other responsibilities, managed to coax an ailing typewriter through the several drafts of the manuscript, as well as the extensive correspondence entailed in preparing this book.

ROGER NEWMAN TURNER
Letchworth 1984

Contents

Foreword

Naturopathy, or the healing power of nature *(vis medicatrix naturae)*, underpins nearly all the therapeutic techniques in alternative medicine. Acupuncture, manipulation and homoeopathy all depend on the body's ability to heal itself if pushed, needled or coaxed in the right direction. Although naturopathy is a relatively recent word, its therapeutic approach and principles represent the essence of a broad holistic attitude to health and disease. It challenges reductionism, which represents the essential philosophical basis and attitude of modern scientific medicine.

Roger Newman Turner has argued an excellent case for the naturopathic approach to health, without being dogmatic. He clearly recognizes the attributes of conventional general practice but also makes a strong case for a more comprehensive and philosophical understanding of health and disease.

Whilst considerable research resources are available to conventional medicine, many aspects of the alternative therapies are poorly researched and inadequately documented. This book does not pretend to provide all the answers, and the author is open about the failures and inadequacies of naturopathy. Yet it will be obvious to all those who read it critically that a naturopathic approach has much to recommend it and should not be lightly discarded. Above all else the philosophical precepts of naturopathy seem to be both sensible and intimately in harmony with both man and nature. Many conventional doctors seem to immediately reject a naturopathic approach as 'cranky'. They should read this book and perhaps they will have a few second thoughts before dismissing naturopathy out of hand!

GEORGE T. LEWITH
M.A., M.R.C.P., M.R.C.G.P.
Southampton 1984

Introduction

There is a crisis in health care. It is not just the financial crisis about which we hear so much, though, in common with this, its roots do lie partly in the technological revolution that has commandeered medicine. Technology has brought many advantages but the expertise and effectiveness which this dazzlingly exhibits in so many life-threatening situations has, perhaps, blinded us to the self-reliant capabilities of the human body in the great majority of illnesses. People's expectations have become geared to reliance on costly and dramatic procedures rather than simple self-sufficiency. But the crisis, like many of those which afflict the body, may mark a turn for the better.

The need for a system that is readily accessible and uses the minimum of resources is now greater than ever. Naturopathic medicine provides not only a simple practical approach to the management of disease, but a firm theoretical basis that is applicable to all holistic medical care and, by giving attention to the foundations of health, also offers a more economical framework for the medicine of the future.

Early Beginnings

Naturopathy is not new; it has been practised from the earliest times. To be precise the first man to rest and miss a meal when he felt off-colour was practising naturopathy; the first people to relax their stiffened muscles by bathing in hot springs, or relieve pain and inflammation with cold water sprays, were applying naturopathic methods; the individuals who first developed meditation and relaxation as a means of calming the turmoil of their spirits were acting naturopathically. Naturopathy is the creation of conditions which enable the body to heal itself as far as it is capable of so doing.

The earliest physicians used their observations of the body in health and disease to evolve an art of healing whose principles hold good to this day. Man was seen as an integral part of nature and the universe, and they recognized that his health depended on maintaining harmony with them. The means of achieving this were present in the basic essentials of life itself — air, light, water, food, movement, and rest. The science of medicine was born when man discovered how these could be used to aid the body in its recovery from illness. These pioneer doctors were, therefore, naturopathic.

This global view of mankind as part of the continuum of nature gathered dust while medicine became preoccupied with the finer analysis of disease into recognizable categories and the development of specific means with which to confront it. Only in the philosophies of some eastern systems of medicine did the whole view of man prevail, and it was left to the pioneer naturopaths of the nineteenth and twentieth centuries, together with the homoeopaths and herbalists, to re-establish the principles of natural therapy. Naturopathy has, in some ways, rediscovered the lost art of medicine.

Basic Principles

In this book I have endeavoured to explore the principles upon which naturopathic medicine is based and to place on record the procedures which are used diagnostically and therapeutically in modern practice. In doing so I may have omitted important techniques, as well as included some others which may not be acceptable to all of my colleagues, but my aim is to represent the full spectrum of practice without imposing any judgement as to whether it is philosophically or medically acceptable. The beauty of naturopathy is that it has diversity and can be flexible within the framework of the vitalism upon which it is based.

Naturopathy has been evolved by its practitioners in the clinical situation, largely by their observation of the human condition in health and disease, and its therapeutic methods have been established by practical experience. It is not always possible to explain how they work, although most naturopathic procedures do have a sound physiological basis. There may, however, be some statements of naturopathic belief which I cannot support with scientific evidence but it would be a far greater mistake to disregard these phenomena simply because we cannot yet explain them. The history of science is full of hypotheses which could only later be substantiated. The postulates of the early astronomers, for example, had to wait sometimes hundreds of years before instruments existed by which their successors were capable of proving the reality of the planets they had described.

There has been comparatively little pure research into naturopathic medicine, largely because it has developed in the clinical situation rather than in academic establishments, and because there is no sponsorship such as the large drug companies offer to a great many medical research centres. Some of the further problems of research into natural therapies will be considered more fully in Chapter 9.

Scientific Verification

Nevertheless, many naturopathic recommendations of the past have received scientific verification, or at least have become more acceptable in recent years. The use of fasting and other forms of dietary control, the inclusion of fibre, the avoidance of refined carbohydrates, the teaching of relaxation and meditation techniques, are all part of traditional naturopathic practice which has more recently attracted greater interest amongst the medical profession. As knowledge of anatomy and physiology develops, some of the theories of naturopathy which seemed rather vague are becoming more refined and precise.

The fundamental basis of naturopathy is the *vis medicatrix naturae* — the healing power of nature — and modern physiology has demonstrated the adaptive capabilities of the body, the role of disease in the process of recovery, and the importance of the immune system in maintaining defence against acute and chronic illness. The measures applied by the pioneers, we now know, were facilitating and potentiating these processes. Even though they may have been explained in different and more simplistic terms they were no less valid; ultimately the success of any treatment must be judged by its outcome rather than its process.

It is, however, by understanding the processes of nature, and the ways in which she maintains equilibrium of living things, that we shall best learn how to achieve and sustain health. I have, therefore, given some consideration to the contributions to the naturopathic understanding of disease, and its often purposive nature, which I believe to be an essential philosophical basis, not only of naturopathy, but of all alternative medical systems based on vitalistic principles.

1. The Foundations of Health

Health is desired by everyone whether it is actively pursued or tacitly expected as a birthright. The use of health as a means of overcoming illness is only lately regaining wider acceptance in the world of medical care, although in many earlier cultures of civilized man the promotion of health featured prominently. Naturopathy approaches disease from the standpoint of health.

Naturopathic practice is based on the recognition that the body possesses an inherent ability to heal itself. Cuts or wounds heal, fractured bones mend, invasive micro-organisms are overcome, and so, naturopaths believe, the healthily functioning body is capable of maintaining a harmonious existence with its environment. This state of equilibrium is subject to certain natural laws, the deviation from which results in disease, and the methods used by naturopaths to overcome disease are those designed to restore and promote the body's own functional ability.

This view embodies a fundamentally different approach from that of modern medicine — different in therapeutic objectives, different in its understanding of disease and, to some extent, different in its view of what constitutes health. Yet, in spite of a practical approach which has made it one of the principle 'alternative' systems of medical care, naturopathy has a great deal in common with conventional medicine and it would be misleading to suggest that they are mutually antagonistic simply because their views of health and disease do not coincide precisely. Nevertheless, in our investigation it will be instructive to compare the established medical view with that of naturopathy and, in so doing, it may become evident that the two systems have mutual objectives which can form the basis of a complementary medical service.

What is Health?

Naturopathy, according to the manifesto of the British Naturopathic and Osteopathic Association, is 'a system of treatment which recognizes the existence of a vital curative force within the body.' This means not simply the action of, for example, prothrombin and the blood platelets in healing a wound, or of the leucocytes in fighting infection, but a less tangible quality unique to each individual and to some extent depending on hereditary factors, constitution, and acquired characteristics. It is often referred to as the *life force*, although biologists have not yet succeeded in defining it. Various authorities, however, have attempted to explore its nature (see Chapter 2).

The concept of vitalism underlies all natural therapies and implies that the ability to withstand disease is directly proportional to the capacity for function of the organism. The healthy body will have greater resistance to disease, or at least the ability to restore itself to normality if it does become unwell. But the manifestation of disease is also regarded as an indication of the body's vital response and not simply the inevitable outcome of infection by pathogenic bacteria or viruses. The organism is not considered to be the invariable victim of bacterial invasion, or other external circumstances, but is capable, by adherence to natural laws, of maintaining its own equilibrium. Furthermore, the ability to undergo an acute illness is a characteristic of the healthy individual — one in whom the vital defensive mechanisms can operate effectively. Measles, mumps, chickenpox, and other common childhood fevers are generally regarded as normal necessities to the development of immunity for adult life. Naturopaths also regard colds, influenza, or occasional diarrhoea, as serving a normalizing process — the response of a fundamentally healthy body, if they do not occur with undue frequency.

Health is, therefore, more than the absence of disease. It is not, as our modern culture has come to suppose, synonymous with hygiene; on the contrary, sterility is the negation of life and health implies the more positive attribute of a biological dynamism. The

World Health Organization, in drafting its constitution, sought a definition which would convey the need of every person to enjoy the ability to take advantage of their potential for vigour and happiness. Health, according to the World Health Organization, 'is a state of complete physical, mental, and social well-being and not merely the absence of disease or infirmity.' Its declared goal of 'health for all by the year 2000' is, perhaps, unrealistic in terms of that definition. We can hardly expect to eradicate all disease and infirmity. Health is relative for each individual and is best measured in terms of a person's ability to realize his maximum potential for enjoyment of life, with or without infirmity.

Definition of Naturopathy

Naturopathy is based on the recognition that the body possesses not only a natural ability to resist disease but inherent mechanisms of recovery and self-regulation. The Canadian physiologist, W. B. Cannon[1] coined the term *homoeostasis* (Gr. *Omoios,* like and *stasis,* standing) to describe the state of equilibrium which living systems maintain when in normal health, and explained some of the mechanisms by which the body responds to agents which threaten its normally steady state.

In practice naturopaths employ various physical and biological stimuli to activate and potentiate homoeostatic mechanisms. They will generally use those modalities which are compatible with the vital curative activity of the body. This means using only agents upon which life depends, and more or less as they are found in nature, such as fresh air, water, sunlight, relaxation, exercise, and dietetic adjustment. Many naturopaths use other techniques, such as herbalism and acupuncture, but these may properly be regarded as auxiliary.

Most of the basic applications act in a very general way on the whole body and this is an important distinction from the therapeutic techniques of conventional medicine. Modern medicine uses a specific and analytic approach to disease. The elements of an illness, such as fever, pain, its location, and blood changes, are categorized to arrive at a specific diagnosis for which there will often be a specific treatment. The disorder will usually be localized to one system or part of the body. It endeavours to reduce the components of disturbed physiology to a definable and quantitative level (reductionist approach). The biochemical changes in the membranes of an arthritic joint, for example, are closely studied, and treatment may be based on some chemical or mechanical intervention to modify the inflammatory process. In other words a disease, or its symptoms, is confronted by the therapeutic action.

Naturopathy also attaches importance to the examination of particular systems and relies, to some extent, on the same understanding of the process of disease, but its therapeutic action is not confined to the part or function which is disturbed. A broader spectrum of bodily processes is treated in almost every case. The objective of treatment is to bring the diseased part of the body into harmony with the whole. This is attempted by promoting the body's own defensive processes and employing measures which are catalytic or constructive (see *Figure 1.*).

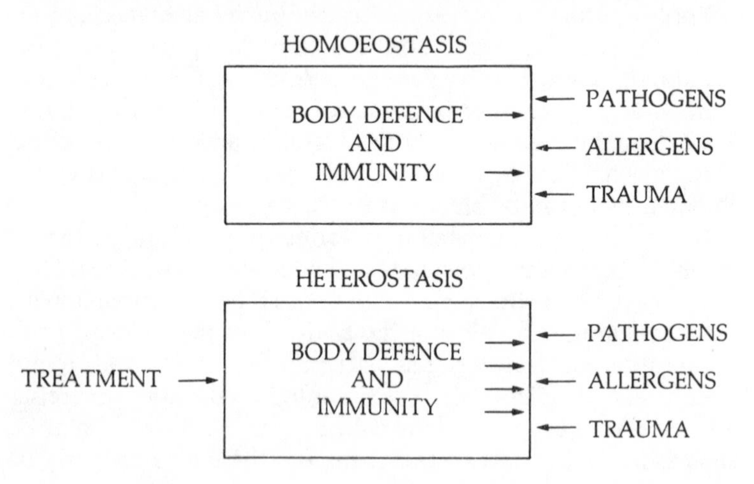

Figure 1. Self-healing mechanisms. In homoeostasis the body defences work in response to infection and injury. These defence mechanisms may be intensified by non-specific treatment (after Selye 1976).

This dichotomy between the reductionist (analytic) approach of medicine and the more general, often intuitive, approach of natural therapy may seem a major obstacle to an integrated health care system. Taken to their extremes both methods have potential disadvantages, if not dangers, to the patient who is dependent on their care. The analytic approach may become so preoccupied with the intricacies of disease as to lose a view of the whole person. The disadvantages of this are seen in the growth of specialization within medicine so that the dermatologist, for example, may be inclined to disregard the underlying nutritional or emotional factors of the skin condition with which he is faced. On the other hand the general approach of some natural therapists may become so bound in philosophical dogma as to risk losing their comprehension of reality. Fortunately there are moves on both sides towards a middle road; the Royal College of General Practitioners are actively encouraging the revival of the 'whole person' approach, and modern naturopathy has a more firmly physiological orientation.

The analytic approach is essential for the study of disease, but naturopaths believe that an understanding of health must be the basis of what Dr Henry Lindlahr, one of the pioneers of naturopathy, called the 'true science of medicine'. In his forward to a new edition of Lindlahr's *Philosophy of Natural Therapeutics,* J. C. Proby wrote:

> If there is to be a true Science of Medicine, it must be, before all else, a Science of Health, and it must recognize that health and disease, like everything else, are subject to laws and are not matters of chance and beyond our control, as is now so very generally believed. A beginning must be made to discover at least some of the basic laws and principles which govern health and the violation of which lead to disease.[2]

Naturopathy endeavours to integrate the analytic and qualitative approach towards an understanding of health.

Vis Medicatrix Naturae

The belief in the healing power of nature is at the core of naturopathy and, indeed, all natural therapies. It is embodied in the mechanisms of homoeostasis by which health is maintained and which is an indisputable physiological fact. But the concept implies some phenomenon beyond what is explainable, so far, in physical terms. It is the existence of a vitality, or life force, which has perplexed philosophers and physicians alike from the earliest time.

Hippocrates wrote of *ponos,* the toil of the body to restore normality, and Aristotle conceived the idea in biology of a life force having some purpose rather than just being. Inflammation, for example, is seen by naturopaths as being purposeful, i.e., a cleansing process, rather than just a phenomenon of infection. The philosopher Kant[3] sought to distinguish the idea of vital force, common in religious thinking, from the concept of 'purpose', which he believed to be necessary for an understanding of organic nature; it need not mean the assumption of a Being acting purposively, although undoubtedly in some fields of medicine, both alternative and conventional, the spiritual influences are highly regarded. Indeed, Dr Henry Lindlahr referred to what he called a 'divine energy' which sets in motion atoms, molecules, and other elements of matter.[4] But he did not believe in the total dominion of mind over body with the neglect of physical reality; rather he advocated a proper perspective on all levels of existence when he wrote:

> The question is not what matter is in the final analysis but how matter affects us. We have to take it and treat it as we find it. We must be as obedient to the laws of matter as to those of the higher planes of being.[5]

There the question of a definition of the *vis medicatrix naturae* must remain, for, although there have been many attempts to identify it, from Paracelsus, who suggested the existence of 'munia', a magnetic force radiating from all living things, through the vital fluid of medieval alchemists, the animal magnetism of Mesmer, to the cosmic orgone energy of Wilhelm Reich in the twentieth century, no one has succeeded in reaching a scientifically acceptable explanation. This may come only gradually and indirectly by studying the laws which govern the body's functions in health and disease.

General Adaptation Syndrome

One of the fundamental principles of naturopathy is that acute disease may not always be a bad thing; it is often seen as the manifestation of the activity of the vital force in restoring equilibrium. It is difficult to convince the individual enduring the torment of a streaming cold, or an acute diarrhoea, that it may be for his ultimate good but it is well known that such conditions, together with many fevers and most of the childhood ailments, are self-limiting diseases. That is, if left to take their course, perhaps with no more than good nursing care, they recover spontaneously.

The physiological processes by which the body deals with threats to its equilibrium are now more fully understood, and one of the major contributions to this knowledge is the work of Dr Hans Selye of Montreal. He postulated that the body responds to stress by a three phase sequence which he termed the *General Adaptation Syndrome.*[6] (see *Table 1*).

Table 1

ADAPTATION SYNDROME (Selye)	
1. Alarm Stage	pain inflammation
2. Stage of resistance	symptom free
3. Stage of exhaustion	collapse degeneration

1. *Alarm stage.* The initial response to a stressor, such as injury, prolonged trauma (e.g. joints under constant friction) or microbial invasion, is usually pain and inflammation. This stage represents what Selye described as the 'generalized call to arms of the defensive forces in the organism'. It is characterized by certain glandular changes particularly in the pituitary, adrenal glands, and lymphatics with alterations in body chemistry compatible with the preliminary attempts to restore normality and heal damaged tissues.

2. *Stage of Resistance.* If the initial stimulus is prolonged, however, a stage of adaptation, or resistance, is entered during which the body learns to live with the noxious agent without the sense of crisis. For example, the initial inflammatory response of a joint to injury subsides but, although pain and inflammation are no longer evident, the friction may continue to take its toll for days, months, or years. An adaptation takes place which may have to be maintained for that time, but eventually the tissues lose their ability to respond and the final stage is then entered which is:

3. *The Stage of Exhaustion* in which there is general collapse or degeneration of tissues no longer able to resist.

Selye called this a General Adaptation Syndrome (GAS) because it is a non-specific response of the body to any demand which is made upon it. Where tissues are more directly affected by stress the same response occurs on a smaller scale and is called a Local Adaptation Syndrome (LAS). The GAS and LAS are closely co-ordinated, for a noxious stimulus to a small area of the body may, in some circumstances, precipitate a general response, for example, an injury of sufficient impact to a finger may induce a total systemic reaction of shock, although local defences should be adequate to deal with the injury.

Healing Crises and Disease Crises

According to Selye inflammation is an active defence reaction and is often, though not always, necessary for the maintenance of health. The response of local tissue defences to infection or injury may be inflammatory, or the more general response of the body may precipitate a fever. Naturopaths refer to these acute episodes as 'healing crises' — a necessary part of the process of recovery. Lindlahr described them as the ascendancy of nature's healing forces over disease conditions and regarded them as being in conformity with the constructive principle of nature. Naturopathic procedures are often directed to promoting an inflammatory reaction by stimuli designed to activate the defensive hormones. Measures such as hydrotherapy, and heat, may be applied to induce an artificial fever, for example, the principle being that the elevated temperature or inflammation increases phagocytic activity of blood cells and removes toxic wastes (see Chapter 2).

On the other hand, Lindlahr classified as 'disease crises' those acute disorders in which disease conditions gained ascendancy over the resistance of the organism. It may be confronted, for example, by an agent to which it cannot make sufficient adaptive response. The pathogens of food poisoning may so overwhelm the defences of the body that death may ensue during the alarm stage within hours or days. Disease crises are all the more likely to occur when the glands and organs have gone into the stage of exhaustion.

Nature Cure

It could be argued that if the body possesses homoeostatic mechanisms and the ability to resolve illness, therapy of any type should be superfluous. All that is required is an adherence to the laws of natural living and nature will effect the cure. Indeed the system of natural healing and living which is described in this book was widely known in the days of its pioneers as 'nature cure'. This term is still used by some naturopaths, particularly those of the Natural Hygiene School founded by Herbert M. Shelton. They rely primarily on basic adjustment to living and eating habits using fasting, dietary management, rest and exercise, but not the adjuncts widely used by many other practitioners, except as short term palliatives in preference to pain-killing drugs.

Most naturopaths nowadays avoid the term 'nature cure', partly because of its rather cranky connotations, but also because the word 'cure' is considered to be misleading. It implies a once-and-for-all eradication of a disease, whereas naturopaths maintain that recovery is a process of adaptation and the restoration of body/mind equilibrium, which can become disturbed again if the same causative factors (stressors) operate. One of the foremost disciples of Shelton, Keki Sidhwa, objects to the term on the grounds that it implies a curative action from outside, rather than from within the body as the natural hygienists believe to be the case.[7]

Nature cure, although still interchangeable with naturopathy, is more appropriate to the way of life which advocates natural living principles. Naturopathy is the system of treating illness which is based on those principles.

The Triad of Health

If health is a dynamic state of equilibrium, both within the body, and between it and its surroundings, it has to be dependent on the balanced integration of the various levels of function, the structural, biochemical, and emotional (see *Figure 2*).

Physical stability is seen to be an important influence on health. Muscle tensions, joint misalignments, or other postural derangements, due to occupational or stress factors, are considered to interfere with healthy nerve conduction and circulation, and indirectly, impair the nutrition of vital organs. Biochemical integrity relates to the quality of the nutrition and

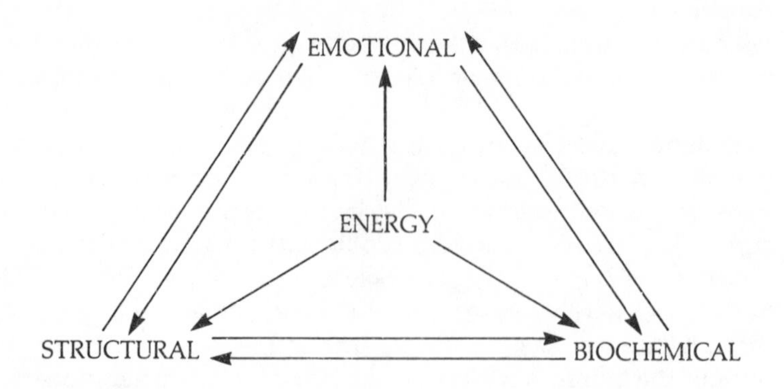

Figure 2. The Naturopathic Triad.

the vital substances derived from food which can affect the composition of the blood and other body fluids. An important part of naturopathic practice is dietetic adjustment and the promotion of 'optimal nutrition' — the best quality nourishment and the physio-chemical ability to absorb and utilize it for the body's needs in growth and repair. Mento-emotional factors are considered to be a powerful force in controlling human health, particularly in their influence on physical and biochemical well-being.

Each of these factors is regarded with more or less importance in any medical system which has based its approach on vitalism. Specialized therapies have developed with an emphasis on one or another corner of the triad. Osteopathy and chiropractic, for example, seek reintegration of bodily functions through structural realignment. Psychosomatic medicine, the study and the treatment of emotional factors in disease, is a discipline which has parallelled naturopathy in its development during the twentieth century, and in recent years there has been a burgeoning of 'mind therapies'. Great emphasis is placed on this triad in current general practice teaching of doctors, but naturopathy is possibly unique among the unconventional therapies in placing equal emphasis on all aspects of what Lindlahr called the 'three-fold constitution of man', and particular importance is attached to the interrelationship between the factors which regulate our health.

Naturopaths not only recognize this mutual interdependence, but consider the basic vitality of the individual — represented in the figure by the word 'energy' — to be the overriding determinant of homoeostatic viability. This is probably what Hans Selye means by the term 'Adaptation Energy'. He regards adaptability as a basic feature of life itself, expressing the view that 'the length of the human life-span appears to be primarily determined by the amount of available adaption energy'.[6] We might add that the quality of life is also controlled by the same conditions.

In defining as their therapeutic objectives the re-establishment of compensatory mechanisms by reintegration of structural dynamics, nutritional adjustment, and constructive psychotherapy, naturopaths would appear to be dealing with the very foundations of health. The principles of naturopathy are, therefore, fundamental to all forms of natural medicine and should be the starting point of all therapeutic endeavours.

In order to determine how naturopaths view the role of physical, emotional, and biochemical factors in governing health we shall consider each facet in more detail, but first, to understand the basis and scope of naturopathic treatment, we must examine their view of disease.

REFERENCES

[1] Cannon, W. B., *The Wisdom of the Body*, W. W. Norton & Co., New York, 1932.
[2] Proby, J. C., in Foreword to Lindlahr, H., *Philosophy of Natural Therapeutics*, Maidstone Osteopathic Clinic, Maidstone, 1975.
[3] Kant, I., *Critique of Pure Reason*, Trans. J. Creed-Meredith, Clarendon Press, Oxford, 1928.
[4] Lindlahr, H., *Philosophy of Natural Therapeutics*, Maidstone Osteopathic Clinic, Maidstone, 1975.
[5] Lindlahr, H., *ibid. p.*24.
[6] Selye, H., *The Stress of Life*, McGraw-Hill, Toronto, 1976.
[7] Sidhwa, K., personal communication, September 1982.

2. The Nature of Disease

Naturopaths consider the health of the body to be as good as the health of each of the cells of which it is composed. Every cell requires for its vital functions adequate nutrition, drainage, and, collectively as various anatomical entities, good innervation. Disease is considered to be likely when interference with any of these basic essentials causes a lowered vitality.

There is little doubt that disease is a natural phenomenon, occurring, as it does throughout the plant and animal kingdoms, although, according to naturopathic theory, it represents a departure from nature's laws. One of the major differences from conventional views of disease is the belief that illness can sometimes serve a useful purpose and need not always be regarded as undesirable.

The 'nature of disease' was the term used by J. E. R. McDonagh[1] to embrace his studies, spanning forty years, of the processes and causes of illness in plants, animals, and man, at the Nature of Disease Institute. McDonagh set out to establish the Unitary concept of disease as the basis for an ecologically based science which integrated its various branches, such as agriculture, veterinary science, and medicine, into a co-ordinated theory. The unitary concept suggests, basically, that there is only one disease and that what are known as 'diseases' are no more than manifestations of the damage suffered by the protein of the blood. The prevailing medical view is that disease has a specific aetiology and that, by identifying the individual factor responsible — for example a virus as the cause of some types of cancer, or a specific biochemical deficiency in arthritis — the discovery of a drug to destroy the virus or replacement of the deficient chemical will bring about a cure. There are, however, signs of a shift in this attitude towards the more complete view of man that naturopaths have always held.

In his *Philosophy of Natural Therapeutics* Dr Henry Lindlahr defined disease as 'abnormal or inharmonious vibration of the elements and forces composing the human entity on one or more planes of being'.[2] These disturbances of our vibrational pattern, he maintained, are due to:

1. lowered vitality,
2. abnormal composition of blood and lymph,
3. accumulation of morbid materials and poisons.

They are an adequate summary of the theories of disease causation which form the basis of all natural therapies. One view, supported by the theories of modern particle physics, is that vitality may be expressed in terms of the vibrational quality of living things; this in turn is dependent upon the composition of the body fluids, — in particular their nutrition — and may be impaired by the inadequately neutralized and eliminated products of metabolism. The latter concepts, with many allied ideas known collectively as the 'toxaemia theories', have held great sway in naturopathic thought. We shall consider them in more detail since they materially influence the type of therapeutic procedures employed by naturopaths.

The study of disease must also include a consideration of hereditary influences as well as those traits which are acquired in later life, and the precipitating factors which may initiate the disease process. The latter may be, for example, microbial and we shall consider the role of bacteria and viruses, since their importance in disease aetiology has a different emphasis in natural therapy from that of mainstream medicine.

Vibration and Vitality

In defining his Unitary Theory of Disease, J. E. R. McDonagh described it as '. . . the departure from health caused by invaders deflecting the rhythm as it describes its cycles in the protein, thus rendering aberrant the changes the protein undergoes'.[3] McDonagh postulated a primordial activity (life-force or energy) from which all matter is derived. This matter exhibits pulsation and has the function of storage, radiation, and attraction. In man and animals this is a property of the protein of the blood which is said to expand and contract. (A complex and variable process of protein condensation was described by McDonagh based on measurements of total protein and viscosity of the blood in his patients over many years. The percentage of blood protein and its viscosity falls with expansion and rises with condensation.)[4] As long as this continues rhythmically the body functions healthily, rather like a well rehearsed orchestra, but if any part ceases to do so there will be manifestations of disease — the 'inharmonious vibration' of which Lindlahr wrote. McDonagh went on to say 'the manifestations of disease may be divided into acquired and inherited, and the former may be separated into acute, sub-acute, and chronic'.[3]

The degree of vital activity exhibited in disease processes is also crucial to naturopathic practice. Acute disease can often be indicative of defensive activity at work in the body and should not always be confronted by treatments designed to abort the symptoms. In the previous chapter reference was made to Hans Selye's view that inflammation is often a physiological defence process. McDonagh gave another view of Selye's stages of response to noxious stimuli when he wrote:

> Whether a manifestation becomes acute, sub-acute, or chronic depends upon the number of the cycles in the description of which the rhythm continues to be deflected. When the rhythm is first deflected the manifestation produced is acute; when it is recurrently deflected, it is sub-acute; and when the rhythm is constantly deflected the manifestation is chronic.[5]

In other words the more acute reactions occur in the alarm phase, characterized by pain, inflammation, or fever, when tissues are making their first active response to adverse stimuli. As the adaptive phase is entered there is less vibrational activity, some tissue changes may become evident, and there may be intermittent acute manifestations. Prolonged exposure to unremitting stressors leads to the stage of exhaustion, described by Selye, and the chronic disease to which McDonagh alludes.

McDonagh made extensive studies of his patients, published a great deal of data, and developed his theory to a complexity too great to consider here, but a summary of his theories could be regarded as a statement of the naturopathic creed. He stated that:

1. there is only one disease;
2. that disease is fundamentally the same in plants, animals, and man;
3. that there are several manifestations of disease;
4. that the manifestations are due to disturbances of the protein in the blood of animals and man.

The factors responsible for the damage — referred to by McDonagh as 'invaders' — are climatic, faultily grown food, and pathogenic activity from developmental forms of bacillae which reside in the intestines. In other words, McDonagh correlates the naturopathic view that an understanding of health and disease are dependent, not only on the study of man, but also his food, the soil on which it is grown, and his total interaction with his environment.

Blueprint for Disease

The quality of health, that is the ability to maintain homoeostasis, depends upon a variety of factors, some of which are beyond the control of the individual. These are the prenatal factors, such as the genetic constitution of the parents, and influences during development of the fetus in the womb. The importance of nutritional, structural, and emotional factors, to those planning to raise children, both fathers and mothers, cannot be too strongly emphasized, and many couples have consulted naturopaths for screening and advice on these topics before conception.

If we co-ordinate the work of a number of scientists in the field of biological medicine it is possible to build a theory of the evolution of disease from earlier generations which may provide the foundation for an effective preventive system. What may be regarded as a 'blueprint' for our understanding of all chronic disease has been postulated by Josef Issels in his theories on the pathogenesis of cancer.[6] He suggests that cancer is a generalized disease of the body and that it arises in five phases, which may be regarded as the origin of almost all illnesses with which physicians are actually confronted. These phases, modified from Issels' conception, are:

1. causal factors, leading to
2. secondary damage, leading to
3. disease milieu and lowered resistance, leading to
4. susceptibility to infection and pathological change, leading to
5. disease symptoms. (see *Figure 3*).

No matter what the final symptoms or underlying pathology, the same aetiological sequence may be supposed. Although recognition of these stages is not unique to naturopathy their importance has largely been ignored by conventional medicine, in which great resources are directed to the intimate study of the last two phases, the symptomatology and pathology of disease.

Prenatal Factors

Prenatal and postnatal causal factors correspond to the inherited and acquired disturbances which McDonagh described. Prenatal factors may include the miasms (inherited residual toxicoses which are considered to be present in every cell of the organism resulting from infections suffered in earlier generations), environmental, and parasitic disturbances. In addition Kollath[7] has described a process of mesotrophy, the slow, barely perceptible, decline in the health of the cell owing to poor nutrition. Environmental pollution is a threat to the child in the womb which is highly vulnerable, especially during the first three months of pregnancy, to drugs, nicotine, alcohol, mental stress in the mother, dietary factors, and radiation. Therefore, the newborn child, in the view of Issels

> . . . comes into the world with a mortgage which is the sum total of all damage sustained in previous generations and imprinted in the genetic structures. There is no doubt that this negative dowry is partly responsible for subsequent deterioration in health and the increase in chronic illness.[8]

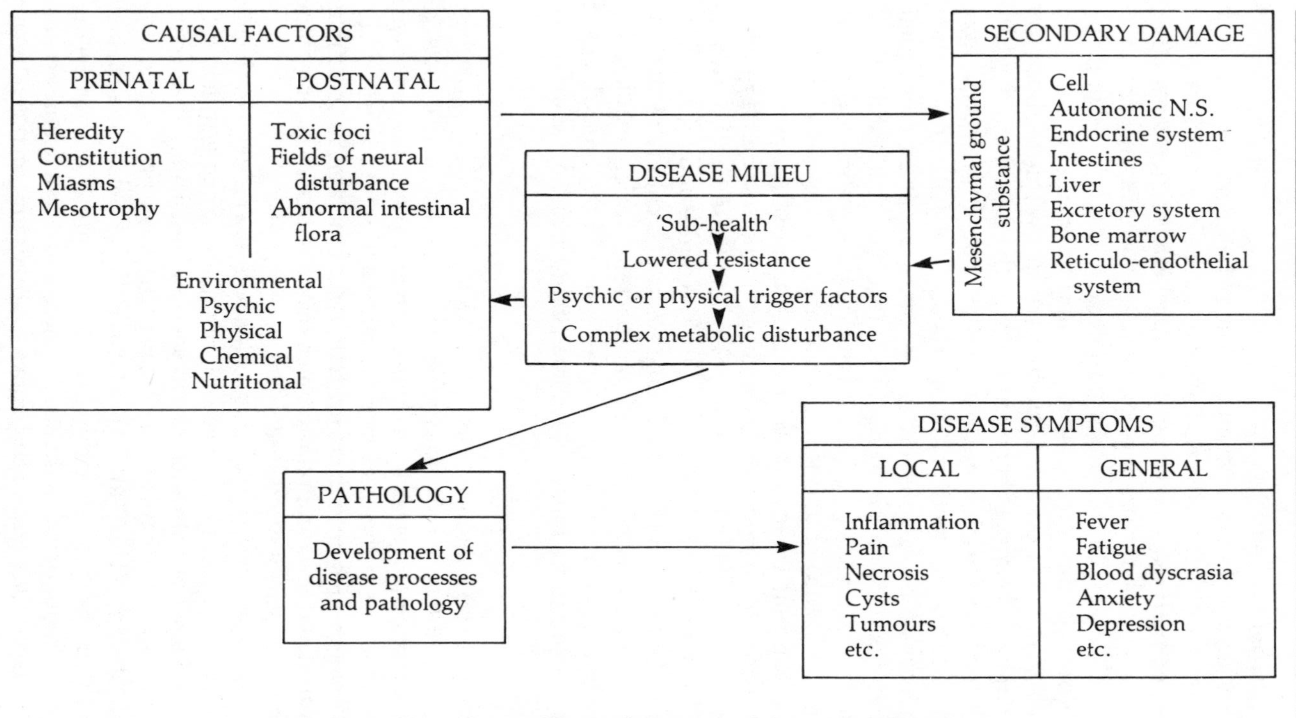

Figure 3. Hypothesis of the pathogenesis of disease (after Issels 1975).

Postnatal Factors

This legacy of toxic encumbrance may be increased after birth by the cumulative effects of various devitalizing factors which can be both external (exogenous) and internal (endogenous).

Exogenous factors include such environmental hazards as chemical pollution (from atmospheric influences and in food), physical traumas, psychic stress, and poor quality nutrition. Endogenous factors are disturbances arising within the body, for example, abnormal bacterial flora in the intestines, fields of disturbance arising from noxious stimuli or allergens, and toxic foci, such as bad teeth or infected tonsils. We shall consider some individual exogenous factors in more detail in subsequent chapters. Internal changes, such as those to the intestinal flora, can be the result of a faulty diet as well as the ingestion of chemicals and antibiotics, but once the imbalance becomes established it can continue to act as a devitalizing agent of some potency.

Before birth micro-organisms begin to grow on all mucous membranes of the infant's organism and these are of particular importance to the healthy equilibrium of the body throughout life. An area which should have a thriving colony of bacteria is the intestines. They harbour bacteria which regulate the formation of healthy stools, play a role in the breakdown of cellulose and assimilation of some vitamins, and act as defensive organisms.

Toxaemia Theories

These are based on the belief that the waste products of metabolism, together with chemical toxins from food and drugs, accumulate in the tissues of the body and give rise to cellular damage which obstructs vital functions. Lindlahr, for example, considered the accumulation of 'morbid matter' to be one of the primary causes of disease.

As we saw earlier, the health of the body is a factor of the health of any of its component cells. Individually or collectively cells must have not only adequate oxygen and nutrients but effective eliminative mechanisms to discharge the waste products of their metabolism. This 'flow equilibrium' of the cells is maintained through the medium of the circulatory, lymphatic, and nervous systems, but between the cells of these and of particular organs, as well as the muscles and bones, lie other unstructured tissues known as mesenchyme, or connective tissues. These form a kind of packing material around the structured organs and regulate the exchange of nourishment and waste products in all areas of the body. Connective tissue performs not only an important filling and supportive function but acts as a sort of agent for the transmission of nutrients and waste products through blood and lymphatic vessels and the major organs. Because of this function it has become known as the 'transit mesenchyme'.

There is a further important function of connective tissue which is its clearing and storage function.[9] It helps to maintain an optimal electrolyte balance and regulates the acid-base equilibrium of the body. The eliminative functions of the body are carried out by the skin, lungs, bowels and kidneys. Naturopaths place great emphasis on attaining optimal activity of these organs to restore or maintain health, and therapeutic procedures, such as fasting and hydrotherapy, are designed to promote eliminative activity.

If there is incomplete elimination of the waste products of metabolism, toxins from diseased tissues, and micro-organisms, they are chemically bound in the mesenchymal ground-substance so that it also acts as a depository. Reckeweg[10] has called this attempt by the organism to live with its unwanted waste the 'storage phase'. In an earlier work[11] he distinguished three main categories of illness as:

1. Excretory events — e.g., common cold, diarrhoea, vaginal or intestinal discharges, abnormal sweating, and eczematous secretions.
2. Depository events — e.g., fatty tissues, lipomas, calculi, rheumatic nodules, cysts, and atheromas.
3. Degenerative events — e.g., cirrhosis of the liver, pernicious anaemia, leukaemia, carcinoma, and sarcoma.

While there is an adequate supply of oxygen, vitamins, minerals, and trace elements the mesenchymal tissues can maintain an effective exchange of nutrients and toxins but deficiencies will lead to impairment of the storage capacity and saturation level may be reached. The excretory phase is the manifestation of the body's efforts to eliminate this toxic overflow. Naturopaths maintain that it is the obstruction of excretory events which eventually leads to depository and degenerative conditions. This obstructive stage is sometimes referred to as the 'mesenchymal block'. The suppression of acute eliminative crises appears to lead to later chronic disorders which are more persistent and give rise to a disease state.

The neutralization and elimination of impurities is dependent on three lines of defence:

1. Intestinal
2. Skin, lungs, and kidneys
3. The reticulo-endothelial system

Intestinal Filter

The concept of intestinal toxaemia is not new, nor is it unique to the naturopathic school of thought. It was first conceived by Dr Charles J. Bouchard of Paris, who, in 1887, published a work entitled *Lectures on Auto-Intoxication in Disease, or Self-Poisoning of the Individual,* and many other doctors and naturopaths have written about the importance of healthy intestinal elimination. As Bouchard's title implies the belief is that uneliminated faecal waste becomes a source of poisons which may be reabsorbed into the blood from the colon. Some people have tended to support this hypothesis but it would be very difficult to prove. It is, however, more likely that sluggishness of the bowels obstructs what Josef Issels has called the 'intestinal filter'.[12] He considers the function of the intestines as an outlet for toxins produced in the body equally as important as their function of removing the residues of the digestive processes.

In all parts of the gastro-intestinal tract there are glandular cells which secrete toxins and a large part of the faeces consists of such secretions with the mucosal cells which have been shed. There is increasing evidence to suggest that the rate (transit time) and volume of intestinal elimination is directly related to the incidence of some degenerative diseases.[13] The need for roughage in the diet is one of the principle reasons for the naturopath's advocacy of a diet of fresh natural foods and will be considered more fully in the chapter on nutritional aspects of health. Healthy intestinal function is not a purely mechanical phenomenon, however, for the role of the intestinal flora, the symbiotic bacteria which inhabit the gut, is equally important.

The *Bacillus coli* produce a number of substances which regulate the growth of harmful bacteria and yeasts, and are responsible for the motility of the intestines. Among the vitamins which are synthesized in the human intestine are pantothenic acid, biotin (vitamin H), vitamins B_1, B_2, B_6, B_{12}, and folic acid, although the efficiency with which they are absorbed varies considerably.[14]

Faulty nutrition and retained faeces will, according to Kollath,[15] lead to a state of 'dysbacteria' which he considers to be a cause of cancer and other degenerative diseases. Changes in permeability of the intestinal walls may lead to auto-intoxication and grossly damage the intestinal flora, which are also destroyed by antibiotics, such as sulphonamides.

Skin, Lungs and Kidneys

These channels of elimination are considered to be of great importance by naturopaths and many therapeutic procedures are directed to promoting their activity. These range from hydrotherapy to breathing exercises and dietetic control and will be considered more fully in Chapters 5 and 6.

Reticulo-endothelial System

The reticulo-endothelial system (RES) consists of certain tissues present throughout the body which are concerned with the resistance to disease. They are cells of mesenchymal origin as well as those of specific organs such as the spleen, thymus, lymph nodes, and bone marrow. The RES cells produce specific and non-specific defence substances.

The specific defence substances are proteases — enzymes capable of destroying protein substances which they recognize as being foreign to the organism. Protective substances of this type are able to neutralize unhealthy cells and pathogenic bacteria but they are only produced when needed by the body, as defence is normally maintained by the serum globulins (alpha-, beta-, and gamma-globulins) and non-specific digestive enzymes in the blood. White blood cells (granulocytes and lymphocytes) also have a protective and phagocytic function; they can engulf and neutralize toxic waste and unwanted bacteria.

If the excretory functions of the body are impaired the RES may become more active in an effort to deal with the additional burden of toxins, but, eventually, the lack of adequate drainage will result in what Reckeweg called 'homotoxicosis' — the unhealthy blood and tissues of the organism which become the basis of various disease manifestations. This 'tissue uncleanliness' is believed to exist in many people who, as a consequence, are in a state of subnormal health (mesotrophy), although they are not experiencing actual illness. The toxic burden is considered to arise not only from the poor elimination of the waste products of metabolism but from potentially poisonous substances accumulated from pesticide residues and additives in food, atmospheric pollutants, and drugs or vaccines administered for the treatment or prevention of disease. The increasing burden of iatrogenic diseases (illness resulting from medical treatment) has been well documented by Ivan Illich,[16] but as long ago as 1938 James C. Thomson wrote:

> Serums, inocculations, and vaccines, if retained in the body, give rise to strain and liability to ultimate breakdown. Until that breakdown occurs there exists a state of what I have called disease balance. This is Carrel's 'artificial health', the antithesis of high level health.[17]*

General illness of the body may also emanate from acute or chronic infection of specific tissues, according to some authorities. Infected teeth or tonsils may form a toxic focus which if unresolved may impair the recovery of the individual. Issels, for example, considers the surgical removal of all infected teeth and tonsils an essential prerequisite to the treatment of cancer by immunotherapy and other biological treatments.[6] Opinions differ among naturopaths as to the advisability of this measure to eradicate toxic foci, but will generally be coloured by the gravity of the situation.

The stability of the internal environment is, therefore, seen to be of paramount importance to the naturopathic understanding of chronic disease, but it is also particularly relevant to the interpretation of acute illness said to be caused by bacteria or viruses.

---

* Thomson was referring to the writing of Alexis Carrel, a scientist whose perception of the need for a more complete view of man and his environment was almost unique in his time. The most complete exposition of his work is his book *Man, The Unknown* (Hamish Hamilton, London, 1936).

Bacteria and Viruses

When Louis Pasteur said on his deathbed: 'Bernard was right. The microbe is nothing, the soil is everything.', he was referring to the long-running debate with his contemporary, Claude Bernard, as to the primary cause of disease. Pasteur had insisted on the primacy of bacteria, while Bernard maintained that the body's own equilibrium was paramount, and that microbes were of secondary importance.

At that time, there was still no satisfactory explanation for the often ravaging diseases which afflicted man, and Pasteur's germ theory provided a very plausible answer which, after the initial doubts, was seized upon by the scientific community. Pasteur put forward four main principles which have formed the basis of modern chemotherapy and asepsis.[18] These were:

1. that bacteria are found everywhere in the atmosphere and are the cause of fermentation, putrefaction, and many diseases;
2. that each type of bacterium is a distinct species and that this species alone causes a specific disease;
3. that a normally healthy animal has bacteriologically sterile tissues and, therefore, that
4. any disease of bacterial origin must be caused by invasion of external germs through direct or indirect contact with pre-existing cases of the disease.

Although the presence of specific types of bacteria can be demonstrated when a particular set of symptoms is present, and those symptoms are generally relieved by steps to remove such bacteria, naturopaths do not consider the microbes to be the primary cause of disease. The success of antibiotics and chemotherapy in the twentieth century, however, has tended to make people overlook the importance of the body's own self-regulatory powers.

There has been a tendency for the dogmatic acceptance of Pasteur's views to exclude any large scale investigation of alternative hypotheses but many bacteriologists have been able to show that Pasteur's theories, if not absolutely wrong, were by no means entirely correct. We have already seen that the healthy body is dependent upon an active bacterial flora in the gut. The interdependence of man and microbes has been clearly expressed by Réne Dubos, formerly Professor of Microbiology at Rockefeller University. Writing about the indigenous microbiota of the human body he stated:

> Indeed it is so difficult to formulate the criteria which differentiate clearly the indigenous from the pathogenic biota that the distinction is arbitrary and usually meaningless. On the one hand most micro-organisms commonly harboured by the body in the state of health are capable of exerting a wide range of pathological effects under special conditions. On the other hand many of the micro-organisms classified as pathogens, indeed probably all of them, often persist *in vivo* without causing overt disease.[19]

Dubos emphasized that while many strains of bacteria co-exist peacefully in the human body, pathogenic organisms will only multiply when its equilibrium is disturbed by physiological stress. Furthermore, the policy of treating illness by the destruction of pathogenic organisms has not, according to Dubos, significantly reduced the level of infectious disease. What he called the euphoria of health officers, epidemiologists, and microbiologists at the reduction of mortality from infectious diseases and their control has

> . . . not yet been dampened by the fact that morbidity rates of infection have not decreased significantly, and in some cases have actually increased . . . The more important reason for the stubborn persistence of infection lies in our lack of understanding of the inter-relationships between man and his biological environment.[20]

It was another contemporary of Pasteur, Professor Antoine Béchamp, who demonstrated that micro-organisms are capable of spontaneous generation in living tissue, that is, they do not necessarily have to be external invaders.[21]

Béchamp even suggested that bacteria do not necessarily exist in their final pathogenic form in the body but that there are minute particles which he called microzyma, that are capable of transmutation into specific forms, such as various cocci (e.g., staphylococci), bacilli (B. coli) and many others. This was a highly controversial view at a time when electron microscopy did not exist, but McDonagh later expressed the view that the B. coli represent a primary form from which other species develop by mutation.[22] The French scientist Louis Kervran has also presented evidence to support the theory of the transmutation of matter.[23] He has observed consistent increases in the levels of certain minerals in plants and animals which could not have obtained them from any external source, suggesting that they were transformed from other organic and mineral substances.

Viruses

An extensive group of diseases, because of their contagious or epidemic character, have been looked upon as germ-induced diseases but no germ could be identified and shown as experimentally responsible for the disease. The infectious agent is generally thought to invade the respiratory tract and, when exudates from this area are filtered by the technique used to separate bacteria from their toxic residue, the filtrate seems to carry the active agents. Under high powered electron microscopy particles were observed which were, therefore, termed 'filtrable viruses'. They are sub-microscopic particles which may resemble the microzyma of Béchamp.

Examples of virus diseases are meningitis, measles, chickenpox, influenza, and the common cold and, although onset of the illness can often be related to previous contact with infected individuals, there are numerous instances in which the disease has manifested itself when no such contact has occurred. As Réne Dubos states that over 150 different viruses have been recovered from man, then many latent viral infections may be present which are waiting for the homoeostatic breakdown which will provide them with a suitable milieu in which to multiply. The naturopathic view is that this breakdown is generally the result of either emotional, biochemical, or mechanical stresses and that only by correction of these can the body effectively overcome infection and maintain a harmonious bacterial symbiosis.

Treatment of Infections

Naturopaths do not, therefore, advocate the use of bacteriostatic agents in the treatment of most acute infectious illnesses. Instead they try to facilitate and potentiate the operation of the body's defensive mechanisms by physiological rest (fasting and dietetic control), applied nutrition, and stimuli such as hydrotherapy.

The ability to respond will obviously depend on the vitality of the patient and, therefore, the assessment of the vital reserve is an important part of the naturopathic diagnosis. In the elderly and chronically sick this may be severely depleted and chemical intervention may become necessary to reduce virulent micro-organisms to within the body's defensive capabilities. Naturopaths would, however, emphasize self-reliance even in these circumstances, pointing out that adequate nutrition and drainage are still necessary to aid recovery.

SUMMARY

The naturopathic view of disease may be summarized as follows:

1. Disease is a disturbance of the normal equilibrium of the body's functions (Lindlahr, McDonagh).
2. This disturbance is brought about by prenatal and postnatal causal factors (Issels) resulting in a decline of cellular vitality or mesotrophy (Kollath).
3. Mesotrophic changes are due to a gradual accumulation of the waste products of metabolism and environmental toxins (Thomson, Reckeweg). Removal of such toxins is dependent upon the maintenance of the flow equilibrium by adequate nutrition, innervation, and drainage of all body tissues.
4. Toxic overflow may provide a suitable substrate for the multiplication of pathogenic micro-organisms which may then be regarded as a secondary cause of disease (Dubos).
5. Most acute disease is a manifestation of vital function on the part of the organism and is a purposeful act towards recovery (Lindlahr, Selye).

It may seem that disease is an almost inevitable outcome of living. Certainly naturopaths would emphasize the constructive purpose it serves in many circumstances. Acute manifestations, for example, are positive signs of a vital response and need not be feared. The catalytic nature of naturopathic treatment, however, imposes a greater responsibility on the practitioner in the assessment of his patient, and the interpretation of diagnostic criteria in practice may differ from those of normal medicine.

REFERENCES

[1] McDonagh, J. E. R., *The Nature of Disease Up To Date*, Heinemann, London, 1946.
[2] Lindlahr, H., *Philosophy of Natural Therapeutics*, Maidstone Osteopathic Clinic, Maidstone, 1975, p.19.
[3] McDonagh, J. E. R., *ibid*, p.52.
[4] McDonagh, J. E. R., *Nature of Disease Institute*, Heinemann, London, 1948, p.13.
[5] McDonagh, J. E. R., *ibid*, p.9.
[6] Newman Turner, R., 'Issels' Cancer Concepts — A Blueprint For Chronic Disease Management' *J. Res. Soc. Nat. Thera.* (1978).
[7] Kollath, W., 'Über die Mesotrophie, ihre Ursachen und praktische Bedeutung'. *Schriftenreihe d. Ganzheits-Medizin.* Band 3, Hippokrates — Verlag, Stuttgart.
[8] Issels, J., *Cancer — A Second Opinion*, Hodder and Stoughton, London, 1975. p.54.
[9] Issels, J., *ibid*, p.61.
[10] Reckeweg, A. H., 'Die Wissenschaftlichen Grundlagen der biologischen Medizin'. *Homotoxine Journal*, 10 (1971).
[11] Reckeweg, A. H., *Homotoxine und Homotoxicosen*, Aurelia Verlag, Baden Baden, 1955.
[12] Issels, J., *ibid*, p.69.
[13] Burkitt, D. P., Walker, A. R. P., and Painter, N. S., 'Effect of Dietary Fibre on Stools and Transit Times and its Role in the Causation of Disease'. *The Lancet* II, 1408-1412 (1972).
[14] Herberger, W., *The Treatment of Inoperable Cancer*, Trs. Huppert, M. P., Wright, Bristol, 1965.
[15] Kollath, W., 'Dysbacterie, Tumorenstehung, Verhutung und Behandlung. Vertrag auf dem 5. Berchtesgadner Kurs fur Ganzheitsmedizin'. quoted by Zabel, W. *Ganzheitsbehandlung der Geschwistkrankungen*, Hippocrates — Verlag, Stuttgart, 1953.
[16] Illich, I., *Limits to Medicine*, Penguin Books, London, 1976.
[17] Thomson, J. C., *Nature Cure from the Inside*, Kingston Clinic, Edinburgh, 1938.
[18] Werner, Weiant & Watkins, *Rational Bacteriology*, privately published, New York, 1953, p.188.
[19] Dubos, R., *Man Adapting*, Yale University Press, Newhaven, 1965, p.111.

[20]Dubos, R., *ibid*, pp.163-164.
[21]Douglas Hume, E., *Béchamp or Pasteur*, C. W. Daniel & Co., 1947.
[22]McDonagh J. E. R., *ibid*, p.58.
[23]Kervran, C. L., *Biological Transmutations*, Crosby Lockwood, London, 1972.

3. Naturopathic Diagnosis

The first impression of a person consulting a naturopath may be of the similarity to any other medical consultation. The naturopath has to obtain information about his patient's symptoms and background with the same thoroughness as a doctor and, as he deals with the same variety of disorders, naturopathic training includes all the standard diagnostic procedures. But, as the consultation and examination proceed, it will become apparent that the naturopath is seeking information which may seem quite unrelated to the problem and he may reach a somewhat different conclusion from that of the doctor. The naturopath is endeavouring to assess the functional capacity of the patient — his vital reserve, or what Selye has termed the 'adaptation energy'.[1] He must determine not so much what is wrong with the patient but why it is wrong, in other words he attempts to diagnose the patient and not the disease.

Because of the specific nature of the conventional medical approach the diagnosis of a definite disease entity is usually sought in order to arrive at a specific therapy. The great success of modern medicine has been its ability to detect pathological change and disease with increasing accuracy. Thanks largely to a sophisticated technology it is now possible to diagnose cancer at a much earlier stage, and the management of diseases such as diabetes is very much more streamlined.

Yet, there is still a very large group of patients for whom no organic explanation for their illness can be determined.

Commonly these patients are labelled 'neurotic', and tranquillizers may be prescribed, usually with unsatisfactory results. In medicine these are known as the 'functional diseases'. In natural therapy they are a very important group which merit as much, if not more, attention than organic disorders with tangible pathological changes. Pathology is, after all, the outcome of a functional disturbance and, while palliative measures are certainly necessary, the underlying disorder of bodily processes must be corrected if the patient is to regain proper health and equilibrium. Naturopathic diagnosis is, therefore, aimed at assessing functional integrity.

A diagnostic routine may consist of three phases:

1. Interrogation to build up a case history;
2. Physical examination;
3. Further investigations — blood tests, urine analysis, X-rays, etc.

While these are fairly standardized for any medical discipline the naturopath may place a different interpretation on his findings. Many naturopaths also make use of additional methods of assessment as an aid to determination of the patient's vital reserve and nutritional status. Among the supplementary diagnostic procedures are constitutional assessment, iris diagnosis, hair analysis, and radionic analysis.

The information gained from these supplementary measures, together with the normal methods of diagnosis, enables the practitioner to determine the state of assimilation and elimination, the two fundamental functions upon which health depends. He attempts to co-ordinate his findings to determine the significance of the phenomena of disease to these functions. Symptoms and signs such as inflammation, fever, rashes, diarrhoea, thirst, or fluid retention are collated, less with a view to arriving at a categorized syndrome, but more as indications of vital response — adaptive mechanisms at work with either successful or unsuccessful outcome. This is what has been termed 'the significance diagnosis'.[2]

Case History

In building a case history the naturopath needs to question the patient not only about his symptoms but how they are affected by a variety of situations, such as weather, time of day, and geographical location. He may wish to know about seemingly irrelevant aspects of bodily function and lifestyle. A preference for cold drinks, or dislike of tight clothing, may carry as much significance as the flushes or fluid retention of which the patient complains. Like the homoeopath, the naturopath gains from such information a picture of his patient's constitution and vitality.

The patient's symptoms have to be set in a proper perspective and related to previous medical treatment. Localized inflammation, or general fevers, for example, may be of recent onset or of a more prolonged and repetitive nature. The crisis of recent onset may be indicative of a healing or eliminative process, whereas recurrent symptoms might indicate an equally desirable 'cleansing process' which may, however, have been aborted by the administration of antibiotics in the past. Children, in whom the vital response is more dynamic than that of adults, will often have recurring attacks of tonsillitis, colds, or other acute catarrhal manifestations, which might be regarded in a different light to the same symptoms in an adult. In the child they would usually be considered as a desirable adaptive response which could be assisted towards satisfactory resolution by fairly direct catalytic measures, such as dietary control and hydrotherapy. In the adult there may be deeper constitutional factors to be considered; direct stimuli may be too precipitous where vital reserve is poor or where the cause of the symptoms has been repeatedly modified by suppressive drugs. In such cases the family history will assume greater significance, especially where there may have been related disorders in past generations.

The health of parents and grandparents is a material influence on the adaptive capacity of the patient. As we saw in the previous chapter, prenatal factors may increase the susceptibility to endogenous or exogenous factors after birth. Prenatal factors, of course, are beyond the control of the individual, but it may be possible to modify postnatal factors, particularly those in the psychosocial sphere. The naturopathic interrogation invariably seeks to assess the role of factors such as work, hobbies, interpersonal relationships, and emotional traumas in the patient's life, since they may be a guide not only to the constitutional make-up of the patient but to his motivation to gain help by personal endeavour — an essential pre-requisite to naturopathic treatment.

Often the patient's individual idiosyncracies are a useful guide to his need for specific nutrients or other therapeutic measures. The need for certain nutrients, for example, may be revealed by the patient whose symptoms become worse in hot humid weather, when lying on the left side, or when at the seaside, and are improved by changing position frequently. On the other hand aggravation of the symptoms by motion may suggest a need for other compounds. Such indications might lead the practitioner to recommend foods known to be rich in the required elements, but many naturopaths may also prescribe supplements of the minerals in a homoeopathic or biologically balanced form.

Examination

The naturopath will carry out all the standard investigations of a normal medical examination such as observation, inspection, auscultation of heart and lungs, palpation, and measurements of blood-pressure, pulse rate and, where appropriate, respiratory capacity. He may not spend a great deal of time on some of these, preferring to concentrate on investigations which reveal more about the patient's vital reserve, but useful guidance to this can still be obtained from the measurements such as blood-pressure and pulse rate.

Observation of the patient's manner and vocal tone can yield obvious information about his vitality, but more important may be the assessment of posture and structural dynamics. To the naturopath the visibly sagging abdomen, or the tight, hyper-extended neck are immediate pointers to areas of pressure and obstruction of circulation and lymphatic drainage, which may be partially reponsible for varicose veins, haemorrhoids, and pelvic problems, in the case of the abdominal prolapse, or throat, and sinus troubles in the case of the congested neck.

Spinal deviations, or vertebral displacements, are considered to be a contributory factor to disorders in many other parts of the body owing to impairment of either nerve supply, or circulation to vital organs. The removal of irritative neural foci, such as soft tissue spasm, is a frequent therapeutic objective and the influence of this on the naturopathic approach to structural factors in disease will be considered more fully in Chapter 6.

Inspection of hair, nails, skin, and mucous membranes of the mouth and tongue can yield further information about the nutritional status of the patient. A cracked or deeply fissured tongue surface, for example, might suggest a need for calcium fluoride in a physiologically balanced form, [3] although this may not always be verifiable by measurement of the serum calcium.

Such observations have been developed empirically and have become an integral part of prescribing with biochemical and homoeopathic preparations. There is, however, some evidence to support Carl C. Pfeiffer's observation that white spots (leukonychia) on the fingernails are indicative of zinc deficiency.[4] According to Pfeiffer, the zinc loss may be associated with albuminuria (loss of protein in the urine) and white banding of the nails can mark religious days of fasting, or the onset of the menstrual cycle in females, as the zinc level is low one week prior to the period.

Whilst taking note of such observations, the naturopath will not rely solely on them to recommend supplements without integrating other investigations or tests.

Interpretation of Standard Diagnostic Investigations

Because of the functional emphasis of naturopathic diagnosis, the ranges of normality for many laboratory or clinical investigations are not always acceptable to naturopaths. Professor Bernard Watson, Professor of Biomechanical Medicine at St Bartholomew's Hospital, London, has expressed the view that measurements which are towards the limits of the 'normal range' (in blood chemistry, for example) may go beyond those limits when the body is under stress.[5] The commonly recommended levels of some nutrients, for example, are not universally accepted, vitamin C being a notable case-in-point. Pauling[6] suggests that amounts far in excess of the recommended daily allowance for adults of 30-100mg are needed to achieve adequate immunity to infections, but his hypotheses require more extensive verification. Vitamin B_{12} is considered to be important primarily for the treatment of pernicious anaemia, but many naturopaths also find it is of value when administered to patients with other forms of fatigue, particularly that based on neurological deficiencies.[7] A convincing study of the use of vitamin B_{12} for fatigue was carried out by Ellis and Nasser who were able to show a significant improvement in the condition of patients who had been administered B_{12} injections in a double blind cross-over trial.[8]

The averages of body chemistry may often be based on the average for population samples in whom there is a high incidence of subnormal health. For example, the normal range for fluctuations of the blood-sugar level during an extended glucose-tolerance test (measurement of blood-sugar levels over a period of five hours after administration of 50-75g glucose to a fasting subject) would not be acceptable in a patient showing clinical signs associated with hypoglycaemic (low blood-sugar) phases.[9,10] Adjustment of dietary régimes in patients exhibiting these transient hypoglycaemic phases have brought about an improvement in symptoms attributable to them, such as headaches, irritability, fatigue, and allergic manifestations (see *Figure 4*).

An assessment of vital reserve, using the measurement of blood-pressure and pulse rate, has been suggested by A. W. Priest.[11]

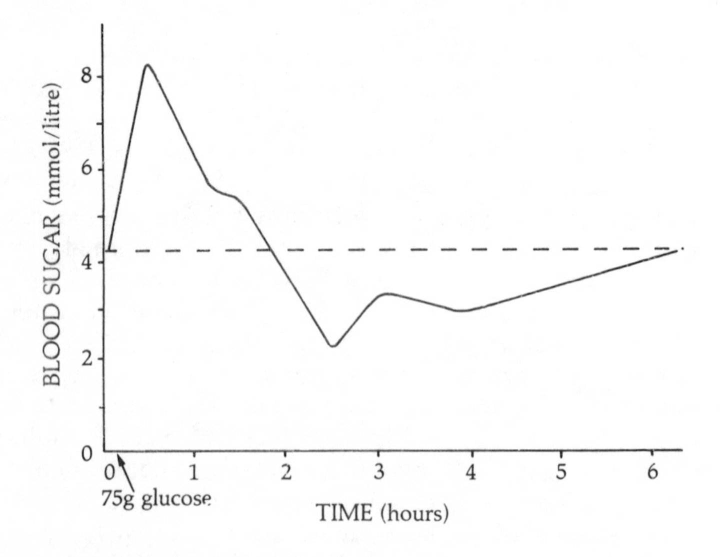

Figure 4. Extended glucose tolerance test results for a 23-year-old female who suffered from fatigue, palpitations, persistent headaches, and overweight. The blood-sugar curve reveals a hypoglycaemic phase two hours after the commencement of the test. There was clinical improvement following the adoption of a wholefood, sugar-free diet.

The Cardiovascular Index (CVI) is the sum of the systolic plus diastolic pressures multiplied by the pulse rate. The normal range is between 12,000 and 24,000; figures below the range suggest degrees of hypotonia and weakness whilst those in excess of the range represent excessively hypertonic conditions calling for anabolic and eliminative measures. The CVI is really an index of circulatory tension, and reflective of metabolic stress. It is, therefore, used to regulate the use of radical diets in the production of healing crises as well as to assess circulatory dynamics.

Biotypology

Although the naturopath endeavours to treat each person as an individual it is, nevertheless, helpful to classify patients according to their constitution (biotype). There have been many attempts to classify mankind according to his physical and temperamental characteristics. Hippocrates (460-400 BC) distinguished between the *Habitus apoplecticus*, with a short thick set physique, and the *Habitus phthisicus*, who was long and thin.

In more recent times human typology has been investigated by Draper, Kretchmer, Sheldon, and many others. The most comprehensive, if complicated, system is that of Sheldon[12] who stated that the constitution 'refers to those aspects of the individual which are relatively more fixed and unchanging — morphology, endocrine function, etc. — and may be contrasted with those aspects which are relatively more labile and susceptible to modification by environmental pressures, i.e., habits, social attitudes, education'. Sheldon subtitled his main work 'A Guide to Constitutional Psychology' but, although he distinguished between different behavioural patterns, the correlation of his somatotypes with disease susceptibility and immunity, at both organic and functional levels, provides the naturopath with valuable additional information.

The constitution is assessed on a simple description of body types such as thin, fat, athletic, or stocky. Sheldon conducted his major study on four thousand male university students of mixed European type who were photographed under standard conditions and then classified according to the emphasis of the three basic components of endomorphy, mesomorphy, and ectomorphy.

Endomorphy means a relative predominance of soft roundness of the body. The digestive organs are large and tend to dominate the body economy.

Mesomorphy means a relative predominance of muscles, bone, and connective tissue. The physique is normally heavy and rectangular in outline.

Ectomorphy means a predominance of length and fragility. Subjects tend to be lean and long in the limbs. In proportion to his mass the ectomorph has a greater surface area and, therefore, a greater sensory exposure to the outside world. The brain and central nervous system are also larger in relation to body mass.

According to the degree to which each component was represented in a physique a score was given on a scale of 1 to 7. Thus 444 is a mixture of all, whilst 117 would be an extreme ectomorph. These physical characteristics dictate, to some extent, the predisposition to disease, with degree of resistance, and the type of therapeutic stimuli which may be applied. They are a further measure of the degree of eliminative control.

Sheldon extended his classification into temperamental components which correlated with his somatotypes. Thus *viscerotonia* is associated with digestive viscera and is the temperamental counterpart of endomorphy. Such individuals show a slowness of reaction, amiability, and a love of physical comfort and eating. The muscular mesomorph is usually more assertive, ruthless, and outgoing, exhibiting the characteristics of *somatotonia,* whereas the restrained, mentally intense and socially inhibited *cerebrotonic* subject will usually be more ectomorphic in build.

These are very broad generalizations and there are many permutations of both the physical and temperamental components of Sheldon's classifications. Few naturopaths make a detailed assessment of constitution by the numerical scoring system developed by Sheldon but they keep the dominant characteristics in mind when determining the disease susceptibility and nutritional requirements.

The predisposition to gall bladder disease, for example, is greatest in those of endomorphic predominance with a tendency to mesomorphy. Rheumatoid arthritics tend to be ectomorphic, whereas those with heavier muscular and bony structure, of the mesomorphic and endomorphic type, are inclined to suffer the degenerative type of arthritis. The longer and heavier intestinal mass of the endomorphs dictate, to some extent, their dietary requirements; they are not so well suited to foods which are liable to rapid putrefaction, such as animal proteins, requiring instead more fibre and roughage from vegetable sources. The 'lean and hungry look' of the ectomorphs is indeed a guide to their need for more frequent nourishment and if they have some of the more competitive mesomorphic tendencies as well they are likely to need protein in larger quantities. Sheldon, who made these observations,[13] pointed out the necessity for more research into these aspects of constitution as a guide to nutritional requirements and this is still much needed, but naturopaths have had sufficient empirical experience to realize the value of the somatotypes in determining the degree of eliminative control which can be applied and selecting the most appropriate régime.

Iris Diagnosis

A further guide to the vital reserve of the patient is possible by observation of the iris of the eye. Inspection is made with a hand lens and some method of illumination, or with an opthalmoscope, an instrument designed for close inspection of the eyes, at which the patient sits while the practitioner records his observations of the magnified iris. Some practitioners make colour slides with special photographic equipment, so that they have a permanent record which may be studied at a later date.

The overall colour and texture of the iris is considered to be indicative of hereditary traits and inherent constitutional integrity. Various other signs represent the degree of toxic encumbrance, both generally and locally, in the zones and segments of the iris which represent the different tissue systems and organs of the body (see *Figure 5*).

Iris diagnosis, or iridology, is widely used by practitioners of natural therapy as an adjunct to their diagnostic procedures, and in Germany some *Heilpraktikers* (naturopaths) rely almost exclusively on this system. They use the more inclusive term *augendiagnostik* (eye diagnosis), since signs in the cornea around the iris are also considered to be significant.

The system is based on what A. W. Priest[14] has defined as 'symbolic topography', and, in spite of various efforts to trace some direct nervous connection between body organs and the iris, no satisfactory anatomical basis has yet been established.

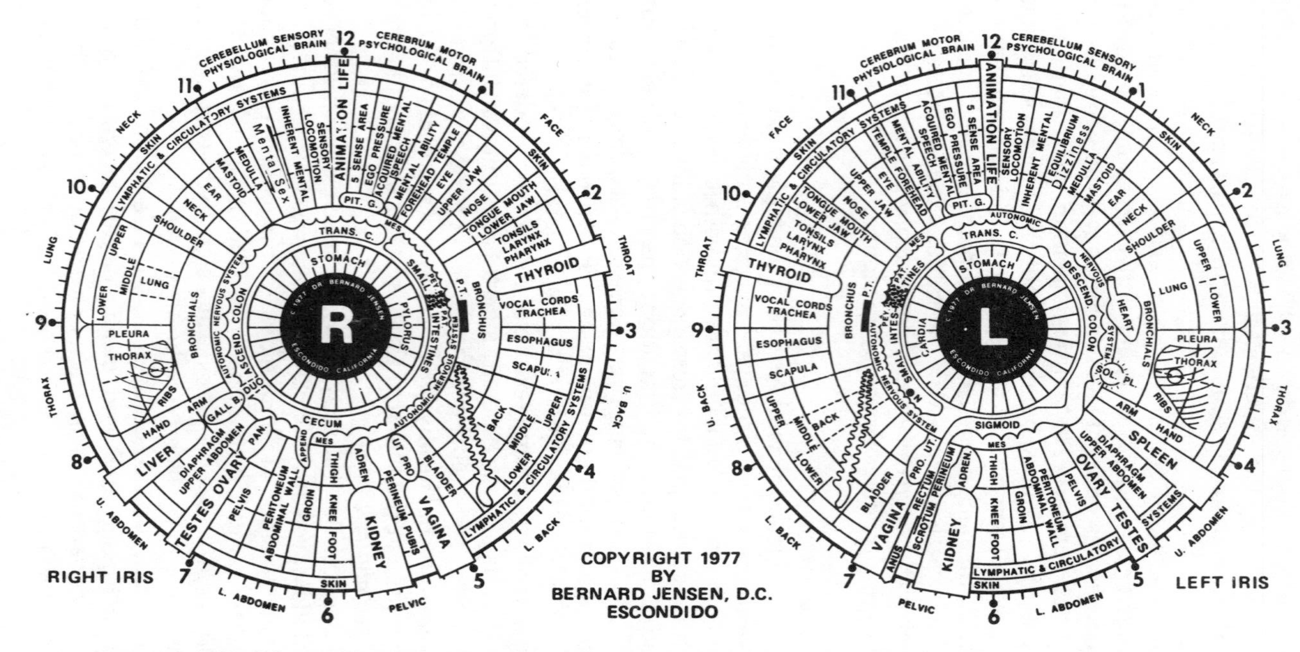

Figure 5. Iridology Chart developed by Dr Bernard Jensen D.C. (reproduced by permission).

Nevertheless, a number of authorities affirm to the view that reflex connections do exist via the superior cervical ganglion, a nerve junction in the upper part of the neck.[15,16]

Priest preferred to regard the topographical signs as holistic, depending on non-physical reflexes. In his view 'the interpretive stress in iridology is upon vegetative values — the indications are actual and only more or less related to subjective symptomatology. The latter merely expresses one phase of failing adaptation of systemic compensatory mechanisms — hence the great difficulty in interpretation is to know what to consider and what to ignore — what is to be regarded as appropriate to the particular typology and what runs counter to it.'[14]

The iris is used, therefore, as a guide to the relative strengths and weaknesses of organs or systems rather than for a specific diagnosis in differential terms. Indeed, the inherent weakness revealed in the lungs or heart, for example, may not have any manifestation as disease of those organs, as we know them, but might suggest a functional inadequacy which would be considered by the naturopath before applying more vigorous stimuli, such as contrast baths or heat treatment.

Iris signs are said to show the qualitative rather than the quantitative state of pathology, although some measure of the degree of inflammatory activity or toxic encumbrance is considered possible by interpretation of colouring. White signs, for example, are indicative of inflammation or over-stimulation and the whiter the sign, the more acute is the condition of the affected tissue.

These are readily observable in blue and grey irids but in brown eyes show only as a lightening of the pigments in the tissues, according to the German iridologist Theodor Kriege.[17] Darker signs are indicative of underactivity of tissues and diminished function. They occur where the superficial layer of the iris has receded to expose the deeper vascular layer. The unnatural colourings which are indicative of various states of encumbrance are said by Kriege to have their bases in the circulatory fluids of the body. He likens these to the yellow discolorations (icterus) of the iris and sclera (white of the eye) seen in severe biliary obstruction and widely recognized in medical diagnosis.

Although primarily of value in terms of constitutional assessment, one study of 640 patients revealed a 74.4 per cent accuracy in the localization of disease when iris diagnosis was compared with conventional diagnostic procedures.[18] Since iris signs are indicative of functional integrity rather than overt pathology, comparisons are unreliable ways of assessing the value of iridology. Nevertheless, Günter Lindemann[19] has shown that iris diagnosis compares favourably with conventional methods in the detection of intestinal problems, heart disorders and tuberculous lesions in the lungs, among others. This would imply an even greater efficacy in the detection of pre-disease disturbance, but clearly further correlation will be required when diagnostic criteria are more widely acceptable in functional rather than quantitative terms.

Hair Analysis

Techniques are now being perfected in the analysis of head or body hair for its mineral content. The technique currently in use is a sophisticated process based on comparison of energy frequencies, known as spectroscopy. Using hair, preferably from the nape of the neck, it is possible to determine the levels of most of the major nutritional minerals, such as sodium, magnesium, potassium, iron, and calcium, as well as a number of the trace elements, such as zinc, selenium, and vanadium. Some toxic metals, particularly aluminium and lead, may also be detected in many samples. Provided the necessary precautions are taken (i.e., unwashed, undyed hair, close to the skin) the figures are considered to be a realistic reflection of the mineral balance in the body and, indeed, some authorities are of the opinion that the hair is a more reliable indicator of the body's needs than the blood, in which electrolyte levels may fluctuate during the day.[20]

Interpretation of hair analysis is still in its infancy and high levels of some minerals may not necessarily reflect a high body level. Indeed the converse may be true as, for example, in the case of calcium. Calcium excretion may be increased in certain states of hormone imbalance in which there is actual lowering of the serum calcium level, while it may be high in the hair. It is most important that hair analysis should be carried out in conjunction with careful assessment of dietary intake.

The ratios between some minerals can be a useful guide where applied nutrition may be required to rectify a relative deficiency of one mineral in spite of apparently normal levels. Zinc, for example, may be within the normal range but in the presence of a high copper level, such as occurs premenstrually, it may need supplementing.[21]

This method is being increasingly used by naturopaths as an additional aid to their nutritional assessment of the patient. Clinical improvement has been correlated with changes in the mineral pattern of the hair of patients under treatment.

Radionics and Radiesthesia

Hair samples are also used in the radionic techniques of diagnosis, although any other sample, or 'witness', from the patient, such as a blood spot or saliva, will suffice. This is quite different from the biochemical analysis of the hair or blood, however, for the witness is used simply to tune into the vibrational state, or rhythm, of the patient, usually with the aid of special instruments which concentrate the energy field.

A number of naturopaths use this technique to determine organ vitality, sites of toxic foci, as well as food sensitivities. Radionics is an autonomous alternative medical system and is mentioned here because it falls within the same philosophical framework as naturopathy.

Conclusion

All aspects of naturopathic diagnosis, then, can be seen to be directed to a total assessment of the functional integrity of the organism — to determine its overall vitality and inherent weaknesses. It is aimed at establishing not so much what disease entity a particular set of symptoms constitute, but what functional disequilibrium they may indicate and whether that disturbance is destructive and overcoming the body's defences (i.e. the 'disease crisis' of Lindlahr) or whether it is indicative of a purposeful effort towards recovery (healing crisis). It enables the practitioner to decide what degree of activity or rest may be imposed on the body's eliminative functions — the eliminative control.

The concept that illness is not necessarily a pointless inconvenience and that it may often be part of the process of getting better, is fundamental to natural therapy. Education of the patient about the adaptive and self-regulatory processes can remove a great deal of the fear and misunderstanding which prevails about disease.

REFERENCES

[1] Selye, H., *The Stress of Life*, McGraw Hill, New York, 1976.
[2] Lederman, E. K., *Natural Therapy*, Watts & Co., London, 1953.
[3] Fisher, L., *Mineral Compounds and Human Disease*, Blackmore Publications, Sydney, 1978.
[4] Pfeiffer, C. C., *Mental and Elemental Nutrients*, Keates Publishing Inc., New Canaan, Connecticut, 1975, p.233.
[5] Watson, B., Workshop on Conventional and Alternative Medicine, Charing Cross Hospital, London, 1981.
[6] Pauling, L., *Vitamin C and the Common Cold*, Bantam Books, New York, 1970.
[7] Pfeiffer, C. C., *ibid.*, p. 158.
[8] Ellis, F. R. and Nasser, Q., 'A Pilot Study of B_{12} in the Treatment of Tiredness', *Brit. J. Nutr.*, 30:277, 1973.
[9] Pfeiffer, C. C., *ibid.* p. 385.
[10] Budd, M. L., *Low Blood Sugar*, Thorsons Publishers Ltd., Wellingborough, 1981.
[11] Priest, A. W., 'Quantitative Biochemical Adjustment', *The Herbal Practitioner*, 5:1, March 1951.
[12] Sheldon, W. H., *The Varieties of Human Physique*, Harper Bros, New York, 1940.
[13] Sheldon, W. H., *ibid*, p.248.
[14] Priest, A. W., 'The Iridological Assessment of the Patient and its Relationship to Subsequent Therapeutics', *Proc. Res. Soc. Nat. Thera.*, London, 1959.
[15] Lang, W., *Die Anatomischen und Physiologischen Grundlagen der Augendiagnostik*, Haug, Ulm-Donau, 1954.
[16] Jensen, B., *Science and Practice of Iridology*, Jensen Enterprises, Los Angeles, 1952.
[17] Kriege, T., *Fundamental Basis of Iris Diagnosis*, Trs. Priest, A. W., Fowler and Co., London, 1969, p.30.
[18] Jarozyk, G., *Augendiagnostik*, Medizin-Verlag, E. Jarozyk, Solms, 1978.
[19] Lindemann, G., 'Von Felke — Prozess Bis Heute — Versuche Einer Überprüfung der Irisdiagnostik', *Methodik und Grenzen der Augendiagnostik*, 13:10, 1982.
[20] Lodge-Rees, E. and Campbell, J., 'Patterns of Trace Minerals in the Hair and Relationship to Clinical States', *J. of Orthomolecular Psych*, 4:1, 1975, pp.53-60.

[21] Pfeiffer, C. C., *ibid*, p.339.

4. The Law of Cure

The self-limiting nature of many illnesses is well known. The common cold, influenza, or gastro-enteritis, will generally resolve themselves in a few days without the necessity of any treatment, other than rest. According to naturopathic theory these are manifestations of an effort to eliminate or neutralize systemic toxins. Although commonly regarded as being the result of infection by micro-organisms, these ailments, according to naturopaths, may occur spontaneously, and can be an essential part of the sequence of recovery from chronic illness.

Henry Lindlahr defined these acute episodes as the 'healing crisis'. They are recognized throughout natural therapy as a desirable, vital response and, indeed, in the treatment of some chronic diseases they are actively induced (see Fever Therapy, page 64). In homoeopathy the active return of acute symptoms which may previously have been suppressed is termed an 'aggravation'.

It was the homoeopath, Hering, who explained the phenomenon clearly in his 'Law of Cure', according to which 'all cure comes from within out, from the head down, and in the reverse order as the symptoms have appeared within the body'. Put very simply this means that many chronic diseases show a tendency to become worse before they get better; the more acute and superficial symptoms, if they were the first to appear, will usually be the last to go.

Because of the general view that illness is invariably the result of invasion by external agents naturopaths also have to reassure their patients that this is not always the case and that their more unpleasant symptoms may be indicative of a turn for the better. They will also point out that the rate of recovery can vary greatly depending on many other factors, such as the patient's vital reserve.

Layers of Disease

In Chapter 1 we saw that the body responds to adverse situations with a sequence of changes known as the General Adaptation Syndrome (GAS). The first stage of active defence, the alarm stage, is characterized by pain and inflammation or fever. If the stress continues a stage of resistance is entered and, eventually, as defensive mechanisms begin to break down, the stage of exhaustion, with irreversible pathology, is reached.

We also considered the theories of McDonagh and others regarding the intensity of vibrational activity in acute and chronic diseases (Chapter 2). There is greater vibration and, therefore, more vital response demonstrated in the acute condition.

Using these principles, we may construct a table representing the levels of disease and showing an approximate scale of vital activity in different illnesses *(Figure 6)*. This may be divided into acute, sub-acute, and chronic stages, corresponding to the alarm stage, stage of resistance, and stage of exhaustion of Selye's GAS.

Acute symptoms, exhibiting the greatest vital response, usually take the form of inflammatory conditions, colds, influenza, diarrhoea, and rashes. Inflammation is described by Hans Selye[1] as an active defence reaction which is necessary to maintain the health. It occurs where any injury or irritant which might be a threat to the body invades. But it may also occur in a localized or generalized form where previously inactivated or uneliminated toxins are mobilized within the body. Henry Lindlahr stated that 'inflammation is a reconstructive process and should not be suppressed. Every acute disease is a result of a cleansing and healing effort of nature'.[2] According to Josef Issels: 'if the organism is unable, or not allowed, to develop autonomic febrile reactions to rid itself completely of the toxins of infection these have to be deposited in the storage cells of the mesenchyme. Residual toxicoses will be the result'.[3] In general it may be said that if the cleansing process does not resolve itself within a few days acute

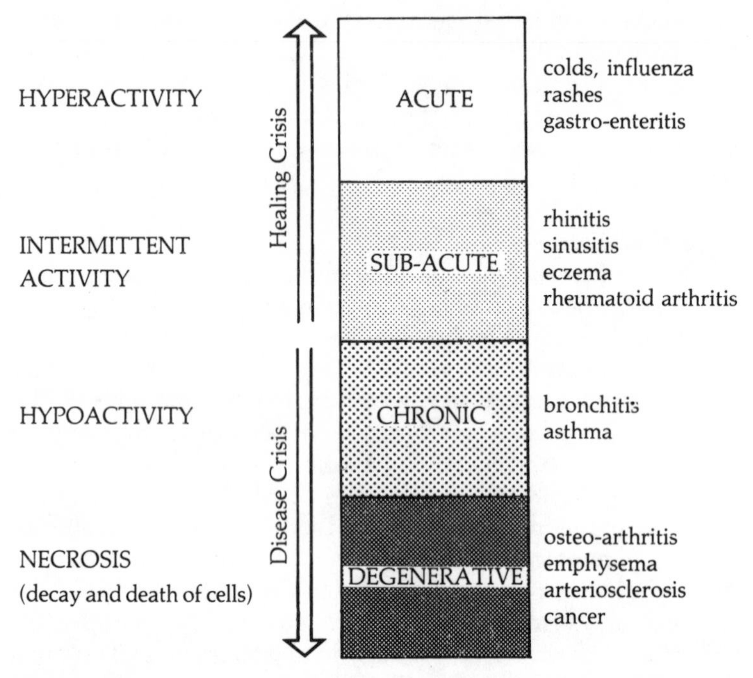

Figure 6. Levels of Disease Activity. Vital activity is greatest in acute illnesses and may diminish as disease becomes more chronic and deep seated. Some examples given may feature at stages other than those in which they are shown.

symptoms may subside into a less acute phase.

The sub-acute stage may be entered where the body lacks the vitality to sustain the level of eliminative activity to resolve the disorder, or where that activity may have been suppressed by a treatment which confronts the symptoms (e.g., antibiotics). The level of vibrational activity becomes lower and there may be only intermittent symptoms or febrile responses. The 'mesenchymal block', which was referred to in Chapter 2 then occurs and the capacity to respond constructively declines. A rheumatic disorder, for example, may give persistent stiffness with only sporadic episodes of pain and inflammation. The colds, coughs, and rashes of the earlier years of life will, if repeatedly suppressed, become the sinusitis, bronchitis, and arthritis of middle and later years, according to naturopaths.

It is suggested by the Unitary Theory (McDonagh) that there is no sharp distinction between one disease and another, and that the uneliminated toxins of colds and influenza can become the mesotrophic foundation for the more persistent ailments occurring at a deeper level, such as sinus and chest problems. The chronic bronchitic may remain in a sub-acute state with periodic acute episodes which are considered by naturopaths to be spontaneous attempts at elimination by the body. Likewise, the subject with sinus problems may experience prolonged catarrhal congestion, with only periodic episodes of sinusitis or heavy colds. As time goes by the ability to respond with inflammatory or other vital responses declines and conditions become more chronic. The mesenchymal block has already occurred. Eventually degenerative changes may take place. Lungs which have become less and less efficient may develop fibrous tissue and become emphysematous (distention of air sacs owing to loss of elasticity).

Reverse Order of Cure

Within natural therapy either passive or active measures may be taken to enable the body to recover. Passive measures are recommended to create conditions conducive to the functions of the body's own homoeostatic mechanism; for example, with rest and by removal of obstructions to normal function, dietary controls, fasting, or gentle structural correction. This is the approach of the Natural Hygienists (Shelton *et al*). Active heterostatic measures are designed to stimulate or potentiate normal body defences — to set the thermostat higher, as Selye describes it. Stimuli, such as hydrotherapy, heat, more active exercise, herbal tonics and alteratives, and nutritional supplements, may be recommended. Whichever approach is used the process of recovery will follow the same sequence. The less active but chronic and troublesome symptoms gradually give way to more acute episodes. The sufferer with chronic sinusitis, or catarrh, may develop a freer and more active secretion and possibly some streaming colds. The asthmatic may experience the same sort of symptoms, but could also undergo an aggravation of the eczema which may have been suppressed in childhood.

These are regarded by naturopaths as examples of disease recovering from within outward. The superficial symptoms of skin, nasal membranes, or bowels are considered to be the ultimate elimination of accumulated toxins.

Naturopathic literature abounds with case reports of people with chronic disorders who have been through this process, but there appears to have been no definitive study showing the incidence of healing crises in recovery, or showing the proportion of such cases in relation to disease crises — those cases in which acute manifestations overcome the vital resistance and become destructive or life-threatening. The role of the healing crisis is so widely recognized in natural therapy, however, that there is little doubt as to its validity. Many therapeutic procedures are, indeed, applied with the express purpose of stimulating such an active defence reaction.

Fever Therapy

The induction of a high fever under clinical conditions has long been a part of holistic therapy. The technique was once known as malariatherapy, or malarialization, as Hippocrates, over 2,400 years ago, referred to the way some diseases could be controlled by concurrent malarial fever.

Today the fever may be induced by hydrotherapy, such as hot mustard baths, or by various forms of heat treatment. It is also achieved by the injection of preparations of the herb Echinacea, which raises the non-specific resistance — a technique commonly used by continental naturopaths.

In the febrile condition the white cell count of the blood is increased and there is mobilization of phagocytic and enzyme producing cells, known as immunocytes. These detoxifying enzymes, commonly known as antibodies, neutralize metabolic toxins released from the reactivated mesenchymal storage tissues. The antibody titres in the blood show a significant increase after a few hours of a feverish attack.

During the fastigium of the fever, when the temperature is at its maximum, the skin is dry and flushed as the body sustains the heat necessary to the increased metabolic activity, but as the temperature falls (defervescence) marked sweating occurs which permits the elimination of toxins.[4] Naturopaths attach great importance to the eliminative functions of the skin which is the reason for many of the physical stimuli, such as hydrotherapy, which we will consider more fully in Chapter 7.

Constitution and Healing

The suitability of subjects for fever therapy or other tonic and stimulating forms of treatment may vary tremendously. The patient must have sufficient vital reserve to make a response and to be able to come through the healing crisis with some degree of improvement in his health.

The naturopath will wish to satisfy himself, not only that the overall vitality of the patient is capable of undergoing more active treatment, but that the various organs of elimination such as skin, bowels, and kidneys, can bear the additional toxic load released from the mesenchyme. The patient's potential for recovery depends on a number of factors, considered below, which may also limit the scope of therapy and the rate of improvement in health. Treatment has to be graded according to the naturopath's assessment of the influence these factors have on his patient's present condition. Therapeutic measures applied to several different patients with the same complaint cannot, therefore, be standardized. Choice of treatment and degree of response will vary according to the diverse influences of heredity, constitution, past history, age, and environmental factors.

Hereditary factors. A predisposition to functional deficiency of organs (organ inferiority), such as heart or lungs, tends to run in families. Presumably these similarities are passed on in the same way as are facial features. The role of prenatal factors was considered in Chapter 2. Vigorous tonic measures might not be acceptable to a heart or lungs unable to cope effectively with an increased circulatory demand.

Constitution is also governed by heredity. Using Sheldon's classification (see page 51) endomorphs can generally take vigorous stimuli whereas the mesomorphic and ectomorphic types have a lower vital reserve. The ectomorph needs anabolic treatment to build up vitality and can only be brought to active crises by easy stages.

The *age* of the patient will be considered with the constitution in selecting the therapeutic approach. In general, children and young adults exhibit a high vitality. In the young there is a higher incidence of acute febrile disorders which can be allowed to follow their natural course without medical intervention. The vital reserve is sufficient to impose stricter dietary régimes or fasting. In the elderly, on the other hand, more chronic and degenerative disorders prevail. Vitality may be low and treatments are, accordingly, milder and aimed generally at regeneration. Rest, gentle exercise, and supplemental nutrition may be used. Reinforcement of body defences takes precedence over mobilizing of active elimination.

The *past history* of the patient modifies the intensity of naturopathic treatment especially in the elderly. A series of unresolved ailments throughout life may have left a residual toxicosis too great for the declining liver or kidneys to handle. Previous medical treatment has to be considered with regard to both the possible suppression of the illness for which it was administered and the disruptions to body economy it may have wrought by side-effects. The corticosteroid drugs, for example, used for a wide range of acute, sub-acute, and inflammatory disorders, ranging from conditions such as rheumatoid arthritis to gastro-intestinal problems, can, apart from other adverse reactions, cause a loss of calcium (hypocalcaemia) leading to a greater fragility of bone structure.[5] Avitaminoses (vitamin deficiencies) are also common after the prolonged administration of many drugs.[6]

Equal caution is applied when confronted with the type of patient who has 'never had a days illness in his life'. While absence of sickness may reflect a sturdy constitution, the possibility of pathological and degenerative changes always has to be considered. Some naturopaths would regard the occasional healing crisis as a sign of better health and vitality than nothing at all.

The general health pattern of a community tends to be fairly consistent because of the similarity of life-styles among the people living in it. The acceptability of treatment and the likely outcome is also dictated, to some extent, by this factor. Epidemics are considered to be due to such similarities giving equal vulnerability to infection, rather than primarily the presence and spread of appropriate pathogens.

Periodicity

As long ago as the second and third centuries, physicians noted the tendency for asthma attacks to occur at night. Many explanations for this have been put forward, but comparisons of normal and healthy lungs throughout the 24-hour cycle have led to the suggestion that it may be due to a rhythmical variation in the width of the bronchial tubes. In asthma sufferers the bronchial tubes, which lead air in and out of the lungs, are abnormally sensitive and their muscular walls contract too much. The narrowing of these tubes may be further aggravated by accumulation of mucus of a higher viscosity than normal so obstructing the airways still further.

Studies with peak-flow meters, which measure the maximum flow of air out of the lungs, have revealed that in healthy subjects bronchial tubes are at their widest between 4 pm and 6 pm, and narrowest on waking in the morning.[7] This variation becomes more pronounced for the asthmatic, causing bronchospasm in the early hours of the morning.

The rhythmical patterns of many bodily functions are now receiving more scientific attention, and the circadian variations in hormone levels, for example, are well known for their effect on health. The rhythmical change in the secretion of cortisol (a corticosteroid) by the adrenal glands may be a possible explanation for the variations in bronchial tube widths which are so critical to asthmatics.

Biorhythms. A differing rhythmical pattern for different levels of human functions is suggested by the theory of biorhythms.[7] In the 1890s Herman Swoboda, a Viennese professor of psychology, noticed the rhythmical variations of his patients' behaviour. He observed that two distinct patterns emerged, a physical cycle of 23 days and an emotional cycle of 28 days. Later, a German engineer, Alfred Teltcher, added an intellectual cycle of 33 days. These cycles are said to begin at the moment of birth, and, according to the biorhythm theory, have two equal phases, a positive phase, when a person's performance is at its best, and a negative phase, when they are likely to be more sensitive or vulnerable to accidents or poor health. Days on which the cycle crosses the zero line between positive and negative are said to be critical days which are even more so if two or more rhythms coincide in their crossover dates (see *Figure* 7).

Although biorhythms do reveal some correlations with physical and emotional states, their absolute regularity does not take account of biological individuality. Nevertheless, as an exercise in the observation of bodily rhythms the theory provides a useful framework for further study of the fluctuations in health and disease.

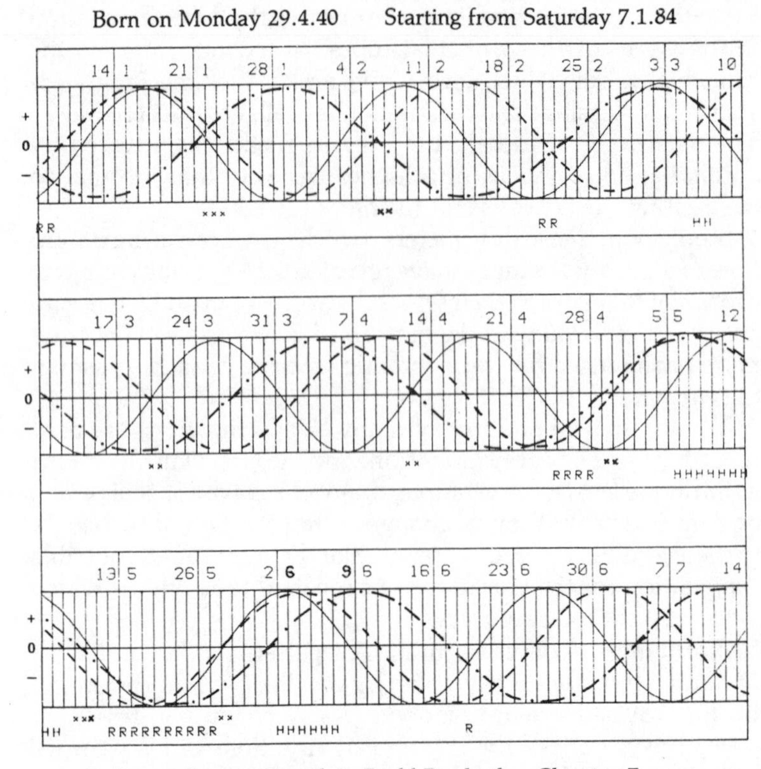

Figure 7. A typical Biorhythm Chart for six months. Physical (23 day cycle) ———. Sensitivity (28 days) — — — —. Intellectual (33 days) —·—·—·—. H = High Activity Phase. R = Resting Phase. Rhythms crossing the 0 line give unstable/accident prone/'critical' days. Days marked XX are critical days calling for extra care.

Law of Sevens. The periodicity of crises in health and disease was noted by Henry Lindlahr, who also observed that a 'Law of Sevens' operated in both febrile and chronic disorders. The significance of the cycle of seven is steeped in antiquity. Traditional Chinese medical texts refer to the seven-year cycles of women's development.[8] Many febrile or inflammatory diseases run a course approximating to one week or multiples thereof, and in the treatment of chronic disease by natural methods

Lindlahr observed the following manifestations of the law of crisis and periodicity:

> When a chronic patient, whose chances of cure are good, is placed under proper (natural) conditions of living and treatment he will, as a rule, experience five weeks of marked improvement. The sixth week, if conditions are favourable, usually marks the beginning of acute reactions, or healing crises. This means that the healing forces of the organism have grown strong enough to begin the work of acute elimination. By all sorts of acute reactions, such as skin eruptions, diarrhoeas, feverish, inflammatory, and catarrhal conditions, boils, abcesses, (and) muco-purulent discharges, nature now endeavours to remove the latent, chronic disease taints from the system.[2]

Recovery Gradients

The initial improvement followed by aggravation of symptoms referred to by Lindlahr has often given rise to confusion and disappointment in patients undergoing natural therapy who have not fully understood the course of recovery from chronic illness. The multiple factors which govern the nature of an illness, the type of treatment, and the response, give rise to a number of different patterns of recovery.

If we plot the level of return to good health against time we can illustrate these variations graphically *(Figure 8)*. The return to health can be considered to have two stages, first the relief of pain and acute symptoms and later the complete recovery, with self-sufficiency and removal of all elements of the illness. The time scale may be measured in terms of days, weeks, or months, and even years, depending on the nature of the illness.

The most common pattern *(Figure 8a)* is seen in the more acute disorders when early relief of symptoms is followed by a more gradual but progressive recovery. In other cases, the initial relief may be followed by an aggravation of symptoms *(Figure 8b)*. A number of such episodes may occur with decreasing severity before there is eventual freedom from all symptoms. A sufferer from chronic bronchitis, for example, may experience some initial relief with the introduction of the physical and dietary measures advised by the naturopath, to be followed by one or more episodes of catarrhal elimination — perhaps chesty colds. These are the eliminative crises to which Lindlahr, Thomson, and others refer.

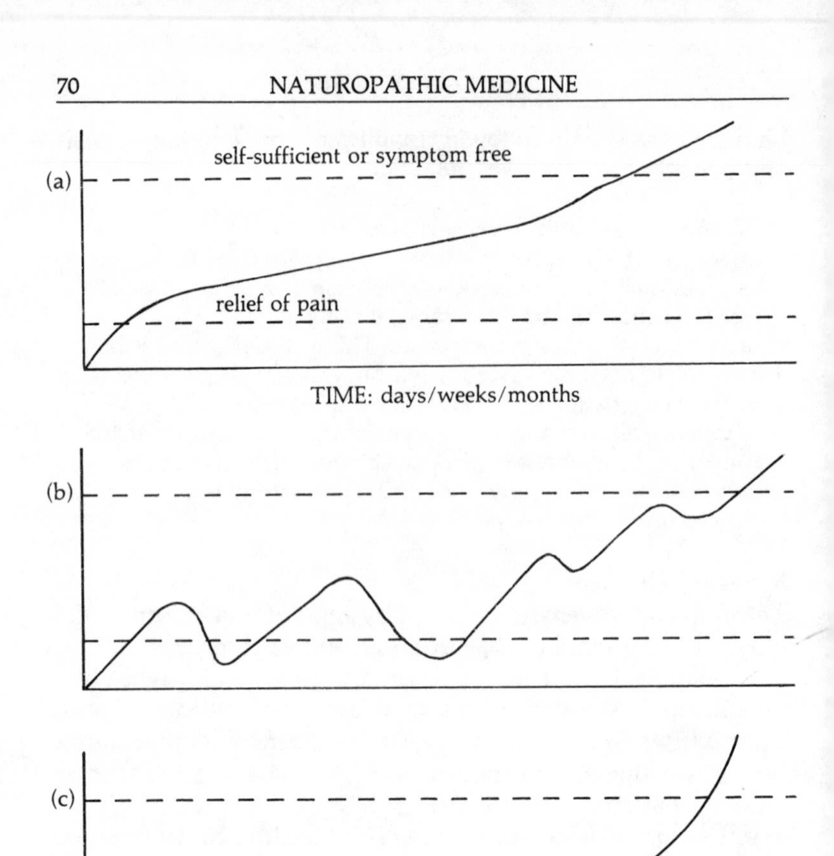

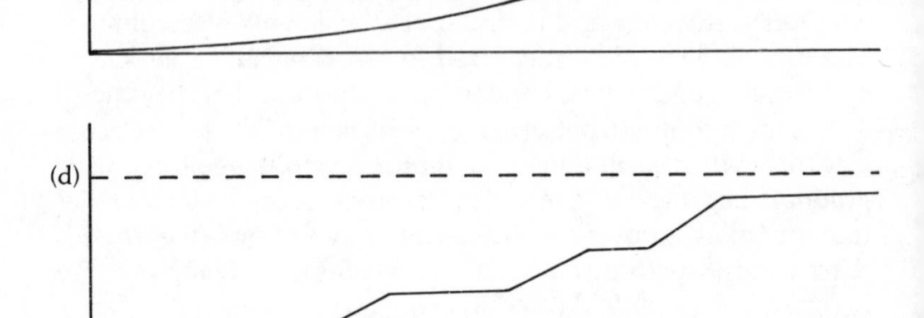

Figure 8. Recovery Gradients.

Where the vital response is poorer, there may have to be a long period of anabolic (strengthening) treatment before relief is obtained *(Figure 8c)*. Chronic disorders of the spine or other joints, as in arthritis, may require a long period of nutritional, structural, and general tonic measures to restore sufficient adaptive capacity to remain mobile and pain-free. Once the therapeutic breakthrough is achieved recovery may be more rapid, or there may be a plateau in the gradient of progress when little improvement occurs. Sometimes therapeutic support is needed indefinitely where the vitality is insufficient to enable a complete recovery to take place and degenerative changes are too great to overcome *(Figure 8d)*. In osteo-arthritis, for example, physical treatment may be necessary at regular intervals to maintain freedom from pain and stiffness.

The limitations on the ability to recover do not invalidate the use of natural therapy. They are merely a reflection of the patient's vital capacity which is modified by pre- and postnatal factors. Naturopathic maintenance seems to minimize, if not exclude, the need for analgesic drugs in many such cases.

A closer consideration of the recommendations and procedures of naturopaths will not only illustrate the way in which they can affect the self-healing power of the body but also emphasize their importance as a basis for all natural therapeutic practice, the foundations of a holistic health care system.

REFERENCES

[1] Selye, H., *The Stress of Life*, McGraw Hill, Toronto, 1978.
[2] Lindlahr, H., *Philosophy of Natural Therapeutics*, Maidstone Osteopathic Clinic, 1975.
[3] Issels, J., *Cancer, A Second Opinion*, Hodder and Stoughton, London, 1975, p.113.
[4] Wright, S., *Applied Physiology* (Ninth edition), Oxford University Press, London, 1952.
[5] Darcy, P. F. and Griffin, J. P., *Iatrogenic Diseases* (Second edition update), Oxford University Press, 1981.
[6] Pfeiffer, C. C., *Mental and Elemental Nutrients*, Keates Publishing Inc., New Canaan, Connecticut, 1975.
[7] Ayensu, E. S. and Whitfield, P. Eds., *The Rhythms of Life*,

Marshalls Editions Limited, London, 1981.
[8] *Su Wen*, Trs. Lu, H., Academy of Oriental Heritage, Vancouver, 1978.

5. Food, Fibre and Fasting

Food has become a matter of major concern to naturopaths in the twentieth century. Dietetics is one of the cornerstones of naturopathic practice and, because it is such a wide ranging topic, this chapter will be longer than those devoted to other aspects of naturopathic practice, although this in no way detracts from the importance of the emotional or structural aspects of health. The quality of the nutritional intake is regarded as one of the principle determinants of the body's ability to maintain resistance to disease and can, in some cases, be responsible for certain illnesses.

There are several reasons why nutrition has assumed this importance:

1. The quality of the raw materials utilized by the body for growth and repair must influence its functional integrity.
2. The rate of change in food production and processing during the twentieth century has been far more rapid than the evolutionary and adaptive capacity of the body to cope with those changes. This has led to an increased incidence of chronic degenerative diseases.
3. Food is the factor over which the individual has greatest personal control.

Naturopaths, therefore, place much emphasis on the requirements of a basic healthful diet for maintaining bodily function and optimal resistance to disease. They also use dietetic controls and applied nutrition to stimulate and potentiate the body's recuperative powers in cases of acute or chronic illness.

BASIC DIETARY PRINCIPLES

The central theme of naturopathic dietetics is that of wholeness. Whereas orthodox nutritionists are concerned primarily with quantitative factors, in terms of calories, minimal daily requirements, and the differentiation of carbohydrates, fats, and proteins, naturopaths, while taking all these into account, are more concerned that food should be eaten as near to its natural state as possible. Quality is, therefore, seen to be the overriding criterion, for the refinement and processing of food will inevitably result in the loss of essential vitamins, minerals, and trace elements, the balance and interaction of which cannot be satisfactorily replaced by synthetic substitutes. The belief that 'the whole is greater than the sum total of the parts' is fundamental to naturopathic thought.

Naturopaths have also long maintained that the refining of many foods, such as cereal grains, results in a loss of fibrous material essential for the healthy activity of the digestive tract. The use of chemical additives and preservatives is also deplored since these are considered to act as cumulative toxins in the body and may interfere with the function of essential enzyme processes. The same objection is made to possible residues from artificial fertilizers and pesticides used when the food is grown. The principle of wholeness is considered to be necessary at every level of the preparation of food if it is to fulfil its optimal biological function.

Unprocessed Foods

Various studies have demonstrated the advantages of a diet of natural unprocessed food in the prevention of disease. The best known work was that of Sir Robert McCarrison in India, and Weston A. Price in various primitive tribes of many other parts of the world. McCarrison noted the relative freedom from chronic degenerative diseases among tribesmen of India when compared with their city-dwelling contemporaries. Price clearly demonstrated the decline in physique of succeeding generations of American Indians, Peruvian Indians, and New Zealand Maoris after western-type foods had been introduced into their dietary régime.[1]

Raw Food Potentials

Over sixty years ago one of the pioneer nutritionists of Europe, Dr M. Bircher-Benner conceived what he called his 'sunlight theory of nutrition'. He believed that the second law of thermodynamics (which states that heat flows from hot to cold objects, increasing the movement of the molecules in the cold) was applicable to nutrition and accordingly stated that 'in a diet of vegetable raw food we find the highest potentials, and these potentials are degraded by heat'. On these principles he based his advocacy of a diet containing high proportions of fresh raw fruit and vegetables.[2]

Many naturopaths and nutritionists have expressed the view that the modern diet, despite an adequacy of calories, and seemingly more balanced in terms of carbohydrates, fats, and proteins, nevertheless leads to a state of mesotrophy — the gradual sluggishness of the tissues resulting in sub-normal health. This is evident by the rising level of faults in growth and development, dental decay, postural and skeletal problems, poor immunity to infection, increased susceptibility to allergies, more constipation, and a greater incidence of chronic degenerative disease. (These may, of course, be due, in part, to other factors such as lack of exercise and abnormal stress.)

A striking demonstration of the biological value of uncooked, fresh food was made by Pottenger and Simonsen in nutritional studies carried out over a period of twenty years on eight generations of cats.[3] The cats were divided into two equal groups kept in adjacent pens and one group was fed on raw unpasteurized milk and raw meat throughout their lives, whilst the others were fed boiled milk and cooked meat. Those fed on raw milk and meat remained healthy, as did their offspring. The animals fed cooked food presented progeny with boney and dental deformities as well as other ailments. By the third generation still births and gross deformities occurred and some lines began to die out. Pottenger also noticed differences in the plant growth in the two runs; the raw food pen showed vigorous vegetation whereas the droppings from the cooked food cats did not promote healthy plant growth.

Biological Quality

A possible indication of the biological superiority of natural wholefoods over chemically imitated substitutes lies in the technique of paper chromatography developed in the early 1950s by Dr E. E. Pfeiffer. In this method filter paper is treated with a 0.1 per cent silver nitrate solution which makes it sensitive to the colour pattern produced when a solution of the material being tested is dripped on to it. A pattern of concentric rings, spikes, and waves is produced, which is characteristic to each individual substance. The technique is used for the identification and quality control of plant extracts in the preparation of homoeopathic medicines.

A series of tests using this technique were carried out by Dr M. Justa Smith to compare the chromatograms of some unprocessed foods and natural vitamin supplements with their synthetic counterparts.[4] She was able to demonstrate, for example, that natural vitamin C showed a more dynamic pattern than the purified synthetic form of ascorbic acid (see *Figure 9*). Similar comparisons were made with wholemeal bread and a standard white loaf as well as various other commonly used foods and drinks. While this does not prove any higher nutritional value in the natural substance, it does suggest a greater vibrátional quality and point the way towards further research into the biological potential of fresh foods compared to those which are processed.

Quantities and Ratios

Although the need for fresh foods is universally accepted among naturopaths, opinions differ as to the correct ratios of raw to cooked food and the relative proportions of carbohydrates, proteins, and fats. Bircher-Benner suggests that 50 per cent of the diet should be raw foods, the main constituent being fruit, with emphasis on the inclusion of green leaves rich in chlorophyll.[5] Chaitow refers to the 60/20/20 diet — one containing approximately 60 per cent raw foods, 20 per cent carbohydrates, and 20 per cent proteins.[6] He draws attention to the enormous scope for variation within this framework.

In the early days of naturopathy it was customary for the raw

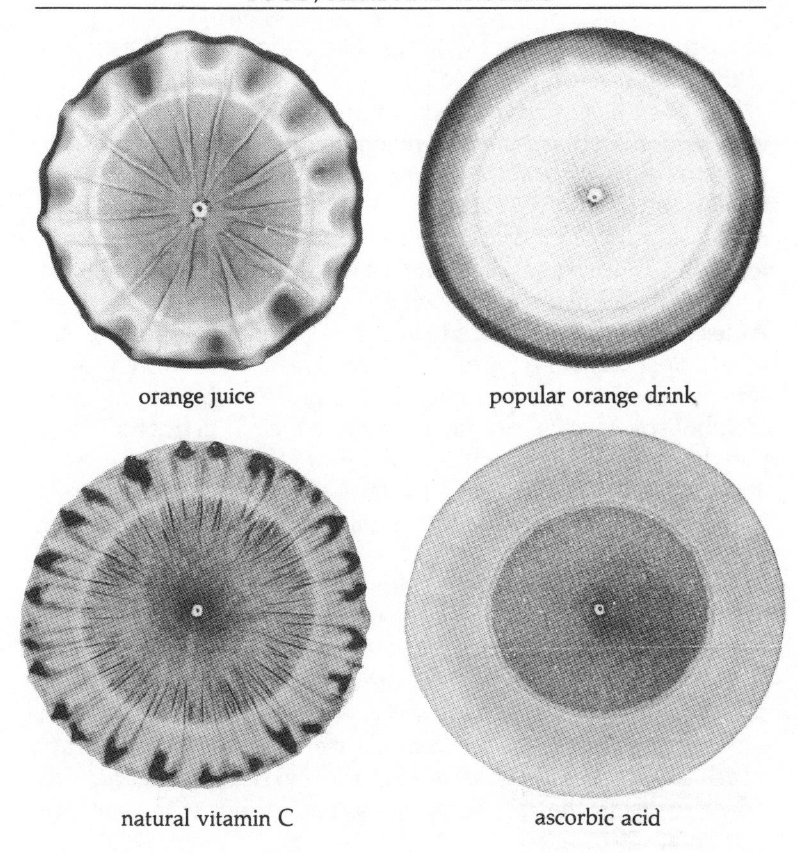

© M. Justa Smith. Human Dimensions Institute.

Figure 9. Chromatograms of natural and synthetic substances.

food principle to overrule all other considerations and be recommended for almost every case. Generalizations about human nutritional requirements have been particularly founded in the analytical approach to orthodox nutrition which determines the 'optimum' amounts of carbohydrates, proteins and fats needed to satisfy the calorific requirements of people in different occupations. There can, however, be tremendous variations due to biochemical individuality and, indeed, in an orthodox textbook of nutrition we find the statement that 'the actual calorie needs of a given family cannot be predicted and their calorie input can be usefully gauged only by direct observation on each member of the family as an individual'.[7]

The basic diet as advocated by naturopaths tends to be lower in calories than that generally recommended, chiefly because of the emphasis on raw foods and limitations on carbohydrate intake, for qualitative rather than quantitative reasons. There have been various reports of the successful performance of athletic feats on a more frugal diet but this would appear to depend on a long-term adjustment to such a régime. When two groups of American students reduced their food intake to about 2,000 calories per day for a period of fifteen weeks their body weight was lowered to a new level and there was a fall in basal metabolism. They were able to maintain their athletic ability but they became anaemic, felt the cold more than fellow students, and they could not keep their minds off food.[8] No mention is made of the nature of the lower calorie diet in this study, nor of its biological quality.

The correct proportion of different nutrients is very much a matter of individual constitution in the view of modern naturopaths. Using Sheldon's classification (see page 51), for example, the longer-gutted endomorphic type is better able to take a higher proportion of raw vegetable foods than the lean ectomorph, with the relatively shorter gastro-intestinal tract which is said to reduce absorptive efficiency. Metabolic variations may also dictate the proportion of foods according to their acidity and alkalinity.

Acidity and Alkalinity

In Chapter 2 we saw that one of the major factors in the aetiology of disease was believed to be toxaemia derived from the waste products of normal metabolism, intestinal fermentation, septic foci, and from environmental pollutants. These are prevented from damaging vital tissues by the buffer mechanism of the mesenchymal ground substance in which they are stored if elimination is inadequate. One of the major sources of exogenous toxins is believed to be food which is excessively acid-forming.

Normal bodily processes lead to the formation of acid wastes which are disposed of in excretory functions, but a predominance of foods such as meat, fish, and cereals may lead to the state of tissue acidosis. This is distinguished from blood acidosis, a serious condition occurring only in disorders such as kidney disease or diabetes mellitus, as the pH (degree of acidity or alkalinity) of blood does not normally show any significant variations.[9]

The relevance of tissue acidosis to disease was demonstrated by F. Sander, who examined the acid-alkali balance of the urine and expressed it as the 'acidity quotient'. This varies during the day but Sander was able to correlate change from an abnormally acid curve to a normal one with patients' clinical recovery following an alkaline diet.[10]

Ragnar Berg was also of the opinion that 'lack of alkaline elements (in the diet) disturbs protein metabolism and leads to retention of nitrogenous substances which cause disease'.[11] This view coincides with that of McDonagh, who maintained that disease was a disturbance in the proteins of blood (see Chapter 2).

The relative acidity of body fluids is determined by the inorganic elements, such as sulphur, phosphorus, and chlorine. In many plant foods the alkaline metal ions (sodium, potassium, magnesium) are bound to weak organic acids, but in most fruits there is a surplus of free organic acids which gives rise to the acidic taste. These are, however, oxidized in the body to leave an alkaline residue.[12] Vegetables and most fruits are, therefore, alkaline-forming foods whilst animal protein and most grains form an acid ash. Foods may, therefore, be classified according to their reaction in the body as follows:

Acid-forming foods: meat, fish, most cereals, eggs, cheese, most nuts, beer, whisky, cranberries, prunes, and plums.
Alkaline-forming foods: most fruits, vegetables, millet, wine, soya, molasses.
Neutral foods: fats, oils, sugar, tea.

There is some disagreement between different authorities as to the acid-forming or alkaline-forming property of foods such as tofu, coffee, and milk.[12]

A naturopathic basic diet is predominantly alkaline-forming. Ragnar Berg suggested that the ideal diet should consist of 80 per cent alkaline-forming and 20 per cent acid-forming foods, but an alternative view that disease is also associated with excess alkalinity is held by authorities such as D. C. Jarvis, Maud Tresilian Fere, and W. D. Kelly.

Dr Kelly's views correspond more closely to those of most naturopaths in recognizing the different dietary needs of each individual. His approach is dependent upon the determination of the metabolic type of the patient which may fall into one of three main categories: vegetarian, meat-eating, and balanced. Kelly proposes that for vegetarian types 70 per cent of the food should be alkaline-forming; for balanced types 60 per cent should be alkaline-forming; and for meat-eating types 60-70 per cent should be acid-forming. The meat-eating types are able to metabolize sugar rapidly and need foods which take longer to digest, such as animal proteins and fats. These, Kelly suggests, also stimulate the sympathetic nervous system and promote the function of the endocrine system. Vegetarian types metabolize sugar more slowly and need the higher proportion of alkaline-forming foods to stimulate the parasympathetic nervous system and the gastro-intestinal tract. The balanced metabolic types have relatively well integrated sympathetic and parasympathetic nervous systems. Kelly stated, however, that the metabolism of some individuals can change from one type to another and modern naturopaths are keenly aware of the altering requirements of their patients. Whilst constitutional patterns may show little variation, metabolic patterns need constant reassessment.

Dietary Fibre

Peristalsis is the rhythmical contraction of the intestinal walls by which the digestive residues are moved on towards the rectum. A pioneer naturopath, James C. Thomson, discussed the far-reaching consequences of constipation following upon stasis of the regular squeezing action of the bowels.[13] He emphasized the importance of a diet of unrefined grains, raw vegetables, and fruit to provide the 'roughage' which maintains intestinal function.

There is increasing evidence to suggest that many diseases more prevalent in western communities, compared with those in underdeveloped countries of Africa, Asia, and South America, may be associated with the lack of fibre in the diet. Conditions ranging from obesity, through hypertension, ischaemic heart disease, varicose veins, thrombosis, gallstones, to diverticular disease, and other degenerative disorders, have been linked to chronic bowel stasis.[14]

Dietary fibre is defined as the indigestible portion of grains and vegetable matter, cellulose and non-cellulose polysaccharides.[15] As long ago as 1889 Professor G. Bunge demonstrated the proportion of unavailable protein and carbohydrate in vegetable foods, and drew attention to its importance to human health. 'We must see', he declared, 'that the diet of human beings does not lack woody fibre, bran, or cellulose. The excessive fear of 'indigestible' foods which prevails among the wealthier classes, leads to debility of the intestinal muscular walls'.[16]

The modern advocates of a high fibre diet base their recommendations on its ability to provide bulk, which encourages peristaltic activity of the intestinal wall. Naturopaths, however, have always recommended that the basic diet should be high in roughage, not only for its mechanical action but because such food, when largely unrefined, contains a greater proportion of vitamins, minerals, and trace elements. The consistency of the contents of the stomach and intestines also affects the capacity to absorb digestive enzymes and the rate of release of available carbohydrate. The slower rate of absorption of energy-providing foods, such as protein, sustains a more balanced energy level and minimizes the fluctuations of vitality and cravings associated with a more refined diet. The non-cellulose polysaccharide lignin in fibre has also been shown to bind bile salts and may promote their excretion. Other polysaccharides appear to be able to absorb cholesterol and promote its excretion. The microbiota (bacterial flora) of the large intestine are provided with an increased amount of substrate by additional fibre, which seems to influence their growth and metabolism.[17] Intestinal bacteria in the colon may ferment some previously undigested polysaccharides and these ferments are considered by some authorities to have an important protective function.[18]

In individuals who are unaccustomed to a high fibre diet this fermentation may create some initial discomfort, owing to pockets of gas, if such food is not introduced gradually.

The Soil and Health

Naturopaths adhere strongly to the belief that the quality of human nutrition is governed by the principle of wholeness throughout the food chain, in other words from the soil upwards. At the level of both plant cultivation and processing of food, the use of chemicals as fertilizers, pesticides, flavourings, colourings, and preservatives is believed to impose an unnecessary toxic burden on the body of the consumer which can gradually interfere with enzyme functions and undermine cellular integrity. J. E. R. McDonagh expressed the view that health was dependent on the quality of the soil.[19] Sir Robert McCarrison noted significant differences in the health of communities in different regions of India which he attributed, in part, to variations in soil quality. Sir Albert Howard made the same observations with regard to the health of animals, and became one of the most inspiring advocates of the organic farming movement.[20] Naturopaths generally advise their patients to obtain food which has been organically grown — that is fertilized only with natural manures or compost free from pesticides — and prepared without synthetic additives.

The forcing of food plants for high yield affects their quality since artificial fertilizers tend to lack the trace elements found in organic manures. André Voisin[21] has shown how the mineral elements in the soil condition the organic matter of the vegetable cell and govern its metabolism. The metabolism of human and animal cells is secondarily affected by the same factors when fed on these plants. It is suggested that the excess of soluble ions of certain chemicals in artificial fertilizers, when they are used, can cause an imbalance of the elements in the soil which may be reflected in the crop grown. Voisin quotes examples of how the use of nitrogenous fertilizers at concentrated levels can reduce available copper; how phosphorus reduces available zinc; and how calcium reduces available manganese. These imbalances may ultimately affect the consumer, whether animal or man.

In one study carried out at the Federal Centre for Research into the Quality of Agricultural Products, in Geisenheim, Germany, the vitamin C content of two varieties of apple, which were otherwise identical in appearance, showed a wide discrepancy which Voisin attributes to the variation in the mineral content of the soil in which they were grown. The variety *Ontario* was found to have almost seven times the vitamin C content of *Geheimrat Oldenburg* apples. The two varieties were compared in the feeding of babies and after three weeks the group receiving the *Ontario* apples had twice as much vitamin C in the blood as the children being fed the *Geheimrat Oldenburg* apples.[22]

Vegetarianism

Vegetarianism (avoidance of meat and fish) and even veganism (avoidance of all animal products, e.g. eggs, milk) are sometimes advocated by naturopaths as the basis of a healthful diet. They are favoured particularly for the higher ratio of alkaline-forming to acid-forming foods. Clifford Quick considered the morphological, nutritional, and moral arguments in favour of vegetarianism and reported excellent results, particularly in cases of skin disorders in patients who had adopted a vegetarian diet.[23] He pointed to differences in the dentition and in the concentration of stomach acids between flesh eating animals and man. Neither the teeth nor the gastric enzymes of man are adapted to a carnivorous diet.

Dr James Williamson referred to the additional burden placed on the liver by waste products and excess sodium in animal proteins.[24] He also expressed the view that meat is spiritually unsuitable for man because it contains 'developed animal soul forces which the human being has to overcome'.

One of the most commonly raised objections of nutritionists to vegetarianism concerns the tendency among some who practise it to develop a vitamin B_{12} deficiency. Vitamin B_{12} is found only in animal products, so deficiency is a greater hazard for the vegan than for the lacto-vegetarian, who may derive some from dairy produce. According to Pfeiffer the folic acid present in vegetable foods may mask the symptoms of vitamin B_{12} deficiency which would, therefore, go unnoticed for some years.[25] Dummer reports several cases among naturopathic colleagues who adopted a vegetarian diet for health reasons and, after several years, experienced various symptoms, including fatigue, weight loss, anaemia, and mild neurological disturbances.[26] These were cleared up by return to a mixed diet. Pfeiffer also draws attention to the possibility of zinc deficiency, owing to the large quantities of phytate-rich foods, such as beans, legumes, and grains in the diet of vegetarians. Phytic acid binds the zinc and calcium in foods, rendering them unabsorbable, but yeast, in bread, destroys phytate, and sprouting the grains neutralizes it. Pfeiffer emphasizes that with careful planning and preparation a vegetarian diet can be perfectly adequate to maintain health.

As with many other aspects of nutrition, most naturopaths believe that the suitability of the vegetarian diet is dictated by individual constitution. Weiss expresses the view that the broad, longer-gutted endomorphic type (see page 51) is better able to derive energy from vegetable foods than thin ectomorphs, who require a more rapidly available nourishment from animal proteins.[27] Any permanent change to vegetarianism after many years of using animal proteins is, therefore, best made gradually.

Macrobiotics

The term 'macrobiotic' (*macro* = large, *bios* = life) was first applied to diet by a German professor, C. W. Hufeland, in the early nineteenth century. Writing about the 'art of living longer' he advocated whole grains, seeds, and plant foods indigenous to the locality of the consumer. The term has come to be applied to the embellishment of these principles with the eastern philosophy of Yin and Yang. Yin foods tend to be those growing above the ground and containing more moisture, such as leafy foods and fruits. They are usually more abundant in hotter climates. Yang foods are found closer to the ground, are drier, and grow in colder climates. They are derived from roots, stems, and seeds. The yang foods are, therefore, said to be more warming and energy giving, being suitable for temperate or cold climates, whilst the cooler yin foods are appropriate to the hotter zones. A macrobiotic diet also includes fish and other sea foods.

From the naturopathic standpoint similar criteria apply to this dietary system as to vegetarianism. The same potential hazards exist with regard to protein absorption and other deficiencies, but with careful planning, and appropriate regard to the needs of the individual, the macrobiotic system fulfils the requirements of a basic healthful diet.

NUTRITIONAL ADJUSTMENT AS THERAPY

Apart from the principles of whole foods for the maintenance of general health, naturopaths believe that specific dietary items, or classes of food may, in excess, be partially or wholly responsible for illness. Equally it is possible to bring about an improvement in health by adjustment or restriction of nutritional intake.

Food as a Cause of Illness

The most obvious way in which food may cause ill-health is, as we have seen, by a decline in its quality leading to a reduction in the vitality of the cell. In many individuals a reduced adaptation energy makes them less tolerant to specific foods such as milk, refined carbohydrates, or meat, the cumulative effect of which may give rise to a variety of problems.

The higher proportion of caseinogen, the principle protein in cow's milk, for example, makes it a difficult food to digest effectively. This incomplete digestion is believed to account for its tendency to increase catarrh and aggravate certain skin disorders. The proteins lactalbumin and lactoglobulin can also give rise to allergic reactions in some susceptible individuals. Although nutritionists frequently recommend milk as a convenient food because, on analysis, it is rich in valuable proteins, fats, and minerals, it does not appear to be so ideal when powers of absorption and assimilation are in any way impaired.[28]

Refined carbohydrates, particularly sugar, may, if taken regularly or excessively, contribute to a wide range of disorders. Because of the removal of fibre, and other essential constituents, in the purification process, these foods are generally absorbed too rapidly. This leads to a situation of hyper-insulinism, in which the pancreas produces more insulin than is required each time for the conversion of the sugar to energy. The repeated pattern of excessive response by the pancreas causes phases of hypoglycaemia (low blood-sugar) which may underlie a wide range of disorders associated with the body's ability to sustain energy for nerve function, immunity, and repair.[29]

Naturopaths have generally been of the view that protein intake is overemphasized in nutrition. They maintain that adequate protein can be obtained from plant foods and that excessive animal protein can contribute to disease. That a surfeit of animal protein may be injurious to health was demonstrated in an experiment carried out by Professor Gansslen of Tubingen.[30] He fed students on a diet of 1,500 grams of meat, 30 grams of white bread, and lemon water. After ten days their capillaries had become thickened, tortuous, and some were dilated and broken. The gums developed scurvy-like swellings and bled easily. More than a month of a strict meat-free régime was required to restore normality. According to Bircher-Benner 'protein combustion in the body produces an excess of acid which must be neutralized by vegetable foods rich in alkalines such as fruit'.[31] He considered meat to be a principle cause of degenerative changes leading to conditions such as arthritis.

Therapy by Dietetic Control

Regulation of the dietary intake is a basic therapeutic tool of naturopathic practice. The patient's nutritional intake may be adjusted according to the need for anabolic or catabolic measures.

Anabolic régimes may be required to improve the nutritional status of the patient where there has been breakdown in their vitality and immunity. This may be particularly necessary in the elderly and chronically sick. The most commonly applied anabolic régime is simply the introduction of the basic dietary plan on the principles already described. Food supplement therapy, the use of foods, such as molasses or wheatgerm, known to be rich in specific nutrients, may also be applied.

Nutritional supplements are a further development of the constructive principle in applied nutrition. Most naturopaths would agree that all our nutritional requirements should be obtained from the food we eat provided it fulfils the criteria of whole food outlined above. They also admit, however, that the diet of modern man is inadequate in this respect and that there is a case for using mineral and vitamin supplements, particularly under conditions of special demand, such as acute infections or inflammatory disorders. Linus Pauling has suggested that the vitamin C intake of man falls far short of that required by the body for defence and repair, and he recommends supplements of much greater potency than the recommended daily allowances (RDA).[32]

Wilfred E. Shute has expressed the view that the diet of modern man lacks adequate vitamin E, which is largely removed in the wheat refining process. He has found that the oxygen-sparing effect of vitamin E supplements can be beneficial to patients with coronary heart disease.[33]

The approach of prescribing supplements, often in quantities considerably in excess of the RDA, is known as orthomolecular (straight molecules) medicine and is becoming more widely used as our knowledge about specific actions of individual vitamins and minerals is discovered. It is a method open to abuse, in that the specific actions of supplements can become a sole reason for prescribing. Naturopaths who practise orthomolecular medicine argue that it should only be used in the context of a sound basic nutritional régime. Furthermore the biological quality of supplements is also emphasized. Vitamins and minerals which have been prepared from natural sources are preferable to those which have been chemically synthesized (see Biological Quality on page 76).

Catabolic régimes are those which are designed to stimulate metabolic change with the object of breaking down maladaptive responses and encouraging the body to eliminate toxic encumbrances. The commonest example of a catabolic régime would be a controlled diet for weight loss.

Diets may be graded according to their stringency and degree of eliminative control as follows:

wholefood mixed diet;
wholefood vegetarian diet;
fruit and vegetables only, raw or cooked;
raw fruit and vegetables;
mono-diet — fruit or cereal;
raw fruit diet;
raw juice diet;
fasting;

with many intermediate variations, for example, fruit and vegetables, with yogurt or skimmed milk. There are also a number of special dietetic régimes such as the 'Hay Diet' and the 'Schroth Cure' which are designed to promote the self-regulatory processes of the body. The choice of diet depends on the constitution and vitality of the patient as well as the chronicity of his disease.

The stimulus of dietary change promotes the self-healing mechanisms of the body, according to Urbach.[34] There is extensive literature on the many forms of dietetic eliminative régime but very little on controlled physiological studies. Restricted diets have been used effectively in the treatment of a wide range of chronic and acute disorders. The most extensively studied régime has been fasting, since it is the most radical and easily monitored change an individual can undergo.

Fasting

Fasting is voluntary abstention from food for a given period, which can range from twelve hours to ninety days or more. Most therapeutic fasts are undertaken for three to seven days. Liquid is taken as boiled, or mineral water, or some fruit or vegetable juices.

Herbert M. Shelton draws a distinction between therapeutic fasting and starvation. He states that 'so long as hunger is lacking the patient is fasting; but after hunger returns, if he continues to abstain from food, he is starving'.[35]

The principle mode of action is, according to Y. S. Nicolayev, (who carried out an extensive study of 140 cases of schizophrenia whom he subjected to fasts of from twenty to thirty days):

1. a physiological rest of the digestive tract
2. a mobilization of detoxifying defence mechanisms
3. a stimulus to subsequent recuperation

Nicolayev attributed the beneficial response in forty-four of his cases partly to the neutralization of toxins associated with the schizophrenic process.[36] Fasting is often used in modern practice to clear the system of food antigens (substances to which the body may be sensitive) prior to testing for allergies. The removal of allergenic substances may account for the beneficial effect of fasting rather than the reduction of toxins as naturopaths have long believed. Both explanations are in effect very similar.

The physiological changes observed in fasting involve a wide range of metabolic factors including amino acids, hormones, and electrolytes. These are the response to a series of adaptive changes at the centre of which is the liver, drawing on reserves of protein and fatty tissue to maintain a supply of glucose to the blood. During the first few days there is a rise in the plasma concentration of branched-chain amino acids, the basic components of proteins, followed by a decrease to pre-fast levels. Plasma alanine, however, shows a steady decrease which is most rapid during the first five days, and falls by as much as 70 per cent at forty days. It is believed to play a key role in the regulation of protein conversion to glucose. The low alanine level minimizes the conversion of protein to glucose by the liver.[37] Plasma uric acid also shows an increase, which may be due to defensive mechanisms on the part of the kidneys, such as a reduction of the glomerular filtration rate and a decrease in uric acid clearance[38] This may also account for the 'fasting acidosis' which occurs, according to Nicolayev, at about the third to twelfth days of a fast. This is characterized by a reduction in the sensitivity of all alimentary systems, hypoglycaemia, and psychomotor depression. There is a loss of appetite, coating of the tongue, and an acetone odour to the breath. This phase passes with an 'acidotic crisis', a corollary of the healing crisis, which is followed by a gradual return of appetite, clearing of the tongue, and improvement of mental outlook.

There is a general reduction of serum-electrolyte levels but most significantly of sodium, particularly during the first week. This is believed to be part of a process of maintaining electrolyte neutrality which is critical to maintenance of cellular equilibrium. After the initial natriuresis (sodium loss) there is a marked reduction of sodium excretion from about the seventh day.[39]

Long fasts of the duration of those which were the subject of investigation are seldom recommended in office practice, although they may be undertaken by some chronically sick patients in residential clinics, where daily supervision is possible. Lengthy fasts were undertaken by some patients in the earlier days of the naturopathic clinics, and they displayed increased vigour, walking several miles a day, after fasting from sixty to eighty days. It is more usual, however, for a fast, where indicated, to be undertaken for three to seven days to provide the initial stimulus to metabolic change.

Fasting is particularly indicated for febrile diseases, such as influenza, tonsillitis, bronchitis, and most childhood fevers. It is also valuable in the treatment of acute disorders such as skin rashes, gastro-enteritis, and rheumatism, and in many sub-acute or chronic disorders such as asthma, sinusitis, cholecystitis, and colitis, it can provide that physiological stimulus necessary to mobilize the healing mechanisms of the body. Fasting is contra-indicated in chronic degenerative diseases such as cancer, tuberculosis and neurological disorders and also in hyperthyroidism.

Physical stimuli such as hydrotherapy, deep breathing, and moderate exercise are all considered to be essential adjuncts to fasting because they improve circulation and promote the eliminative functions of the lungs and skin.

Guelpa Fast

Long fasts may often be impossible or inadvisable and there are many modifications and shorter versions. The Saline fast, often associated with the French physician Dr Guelpa, relies on an initial loading dose of saline to intensify its action. The first day commences with a teaspoonful of Epsom salts dissolved in lukewarm water. For the remainder of the day, warm water with a slice of lemon and honey, or vegetable broth are taken. On the second day a further dose of Epsom salts is followed by fruit juices and, in the evening, a thick vegetable soup with two thin slices of dry wholemeal toast. The third day is a dry day with no liquid permitted until 6 pm, and then only a glass of dry white wine, which is repeated at 9 pm. Only dry toast or biscuits are eaten with the possible addition of a baked potato. This régime must be followed by one or more days on light salads, fruit, and yogurt.

The saline fast is said to be particularly applicable to diseases of the connective tissues such as rheumatic disorders. The combination of a high saline intake with limited fluid has a powerful cleansing effect.[40]

The Schroth Cure

This treatment régime is also applied to provide a strong stimulus to the metabolism and to promote skin elimination.[41] The purpose of the diet is to reduce fluid intake and 'dry days' are alternated with 'liquid days', during which cold packs (see Chapter 7 on hydrotherapy) are applied to stimulate the skin activity. A typical régime might be as follows:

First Day — dry toast or semi-stale rolls until midday. Oatmeal or rice porridge. 4 pm onwards — 100cc warm dry wine or apple juice. Rice or barley gruel. Cold pack at night.
Second Day — toast or dry biscuits until midday. Porridge with apple sauce. 4 pm onwards — 500cc herb tea, fruit juice, or wine. Cold pack.
Third Day — toast, dried prunes, or baked jacket potato. Lemon slices if very thirsty.

This cycle is repeated for a period of two to three weeks.

The indications for the Schroth Cure are fluid retention and effusions (especially those of rheumatoid arthritis) catarrh, and chronic skin conditions. There are few published assessments of the efficacy of the Schroth Cure, although there are many reports of its successful outcome, particularly from German clinics specializing in the treatment.

Hay Diet

Utilizing the principle of acid-forming and alkaline-forming foods (see page 78), W. H. Hay evolved a dietary system which was a distillation of the knowledge of various eminent nutritionists of the day, such as Lindlahr, Shelton, Kellogg, and Arbuthnot Lane. The Hay Diet, as it became known, advocates care in the combination of foods which require different conditions for digestion.

Proteins, for example, require acid secretions for their digestion, which starts in the stomach and continues in the intestines. Carbohydrates, however, require alkaline secretions, which begin in the mouth and continue in the intestines. A mixture of protein and starch in the same meal is, therefore, contra-indicated because it is maintained that one prevents the proper digestion of the other. Another incompatible combination is starch with acid fruit.

Hay advocated a diet of 20 per cent acid-forming and 80 per cent alkaline-forming foods, maintaining that the selection of compatible food categories in any single meal would prevent the progressive acid saturation which leads to ill-health.[42] Although this system was recommended as a way of eating on a permanent basis it is used therapeutically in the management of disorders of the gastro-intestinal system, where incompatible food combinations can be an unnecessary stress on a poorly functioning digestive system.

Mono-diets

Another form of dietetic stimulus is the restriction of the patient's intake to one type of food for a number of days. This has the effect of saturating the system with the particular nutrients of which the food is composed.

The Milk Diet enjoyed a considerable vogue for some time since it was believed that the protein, fat, and mineral content of cow's milk provided valuable nutrients in an easily digestible form. Milk was given exclusively throughout the day, or in combination with sweet fruits or mineral water. It was said to be of value in cases of fatigue, wasting diseases, and peptic ulceration. Many people with skin diseases, catarrhal problems, and other so-called 'allergic' disorders, however, show an intolerance of cow's milk. Milk has also lost favour because of its implication as a cause of atherosclerosis which may result in coronary heart disease.[43]

The best known fruit mono-diet is the *Grape Cure* in which the patient may eat up to six pounds a day of the fruit. Liquid intake may be limited to water, or grape or apple juice. The treatment is said to be particularly effective for high blood-pressure, cardiac failure, and general fluid retention, a benefit which may be due to the high potassium content of the grapes.

The *rice diet* consists almost exclusively of boiled rice. Two hundred and fifty to three hundred grams of rice is given daily, boiled or steamed in water. Some fruit and limited amounts of liquid are allowed. The diet may be supplemented with other grains such as millet. It is used for cardiovascular disorders and obesity.

Some mono-diets are effective in promoting diuresis and weight loss. The modification of metabolic processes may act as a powerful stimulant to the removal of catabolic wastes.

Selection of Dietary Stimulus

The choice of dietetic stimulus may vary considerably according to the preference and experience of the practitioner. There have been no comparative studies of the efficacy of different forms of therapeutic dietary régimes, and selection depends very much on the vitality and constitution of the patient as well as the chronicity of his complaint. In most cases the patient would be prepared for régimes such as the Grape Cure by a general reform diet for some weeks. Raw food days or fruit days may be recommended before introducing a fast, or other restricted catabolic régime. The non-specific nature of nutritional therapy is emphasized by the fact that different dietary programmes have proved effective in different patients with similar illnesses. The precise nature of the diet would appear to be less important than the stimulus to the self-regulatory mechanisms of the body. Certainly the diversity of successful dietary therapies has made them very difficult to evaluate and this is a field in which carefully planned research projects are urgently needed.

Food Allergy

The term 'allergy' is falling into misuse as people attribute a wide range of bodily disorders to reactions to various foods and environmental agents. Strictly speaking, an allergic disorder is one demonstrably attributable to an immune response by the body to a foreign protein. There are a wide range of disorders the clinical features of which suggest an allergic response but the immunological basis of which cannot be established.[44] These may be more properly described as sensitivity or intolerance to foods or chemicals.

Naturopaths have long maintained that certain foods and environmental toxins are important factors in the aetiology of disease, both physical and mental. The cumulative damage inflicted by refined, or over-concentrated foods, such as sugar, white flour, and even more 'natural' foods such as milk or eggs, in large quantities, was pointed out by authorities such as Lief, Saxon, Thomson, and Shelton. The gradual breakdown of adaptive response in the body leads to an eventual intolerance of the offending food, so that even a small quantity may illicit unpleasant symptoms, ranging from catarrhal and skin disorders to irritability and depression.

In recent years a wider interest has been taken in the detection and treatment of food allergies, a study which has become known as Clinical Ecology. The determination of specific antigens is made by placing the patient on a fast, or exclusion diet from which all possible suspect foods have been eliminated, followed by a gradual re-introduction of such foods by way of a 'challenge'.

The fast, or exclusion diet, if of sufficient duration (usually 3-5 days), allows the body to eliminate residues of offending foods. There will generally be a remission of allergic symptoms which may only return when the triggering food is re-introduced.

A study of thirteen children with severe chronic eczema carried out in the paediatric clinic of Parma University, Italy, for example, revealed sensitivity to eggs in eleven of them; to milk in eleven; and to fish in two. A diet eliminating these foods resulted in complete remission of skin symptoms in twelve of the thirteen children.[45]

Mackarness has suggested that many symptom complexes, including psychiatric disorders, may be due to adverse reactions to common foods, such as wheat, milk, eggs, and sugar.[46] He advocated what he called a 'stone-age diet' of whole grains, vegetables, fruit, lean meats, and fish — precisely the type of régime recommended for so long by naturopaths.

Avoidance of specific food allergens, if determined, will undoubtedly alleviate many symptoms, but some individuals may become sensitive to a wide range of substances which may impose severe restrictions on an already inadequate diet. Naturopaths generally favour a non-specific approach with the object of correcting the basic metabolic and functional deficiencies which are responsible for the breakdown of defensive mechanisms. M. L. Budd, for example, has suggested that many disorders, commonly supposed to be antigen-induced, may, in fact, be primarily due to a chronic hypoglycaemia.[47] By placing undue emphasis on the role of food allergens the individual may neglect the real structural and emotional factors responsible for symptoms.

Cytotoxic Food Test

A new technique of food allergy determination can be carried out on a blood sample from the patient, who then need play no further part in the test. The cytotoxic test is based on the fact that a type of white blood cell, known as the polymorphonuclear leukocyte will undergo certain morphological changes when incubated with a solution of the unsuitable food.

The accuracy of the test depends on the skilled observation of a trained technician but it is being refined and may prove to be a more reliable, if rather costly, method of detecting food allergies. Some naturopaths are using this test experimentally in cases which prove resistant to more traditional methods of diagnosis.

How Much Change?

To some people the prospect of making even small changes to the dietary habits of a lifetime may seem too daunting, but most people who are unwell are happy to feel that there is something that they can do personally to help themselves towards recovery.

Advice to the patient has to be suited to their social and

economic circumstances. Unrefined and unadulterated foods are by no means widely available at the sort of prices that the mass of lower wage-earners can afford and, even in the health food stores, one cannot be certain that all the ingredients are from organically grown produce. Nevertheless, there are signs of a change towards the basic dietary recommendations of the naturopaths, with supermarkets now stocking many wholefood products such as wholemeal bread and brown rice. There are also a number of wholefood co-operatives and shops where it is possible to purchase, in bulk, basic foods, such as grains and pulses, at economic prices.

Important though it may be as one of the foundations of health, the naturopath may, in some cases, make no suggestions about an individuals diet. There is more and more confusing and contradictory evidence about the benefits of, or the harm inflicted by specific foods, but possibly the only certain danger exists in obsession and anxiety about what we eat. Even the most nutritious diet available will be of little value to a person whose postural alignment or emotional well-being are under constant siege through physical or psychological abuse.

REFERENCES

[1] Price, Weston. A., *Nutrition and Physical Degeneration*, Published by author, Redlands, California, 1949.

[2] Bircher-Benner, M., *Prevention of Incurable Disease*, James Clark & Co., London, 1959.

[3] Pottenger, F. M. and Simonsen, D. G., 'Heat Labile Factors Necessary for Proper Growth and Development of Cats', *J. Lab. & Clin. Med.* 25:6, St Louis, 1939.

[4] Justa Smith, M., 'Further Research into a Chromatographic Technique for Vitamin Analysis', *Human Dimensions* 2:1, Spring 1973.

[5] Bircher-Benner, M., *ibid*, p.85.

[6] Chaitow, L., *Naturopathy*, leaflet issued by Friends of the Healing Research Trust, Plymouth.

[7] Mottram, V. H. and Graham, G., *Hutchison's Food and the Principles of Dietetics* (Eleventh edition), p.59, E. Arnold Limited,, London, 1955.

[8] Mottram, V. H. and Graham, G., *ibid*, p.49.
[9] Dummer, T. G., 'The Evolution of Pathological Patterns and their Effect on Subsequent Therapeutic Considerations', *Proceedings of Res. Soc. Nat. Thera. Symposium*, 1959.
[10] Sander, F., quoted in Ledermann, E. K., *Natural Therapy*, Watts & Co., London, 1953.
[11] Berg, R., quoted in Ledermann, E.K. *ibid.*
[12] Kuiper, S., 'Acid Base Balance', *Brit. Nat. J.* 11:9, 1982, p.337.
[13] Thomson, J. C., *Constipation and Civilisation*, Thorsons Publishers, London, 1943.
[14] Trowell, H. C., 'Recent Developments in Dietary Fibre Hypotheses', *Third Kellog Symposium on Dietary Fibre*, J. Libbey & Co., London, 1978, p.3.
[15] Southgate, D. A. T., 'Definition, Analysis, and Properties of Dietary Fibre', *Third Kellog Symposium on Dietary Fibre*, J. Libbey & Co., London, 1978, p.9.
[16] Bunge, G., quoted in Waerland, A., *In the Cauldron of Disease*, A. G. Berry, London, 1934, p.284.
[17] Southgate, D. A. T., *ibid*, p.17.
[18] Herberger, W., *Treatment of Inoperable Cancer*, Wright & Sons, Bristol, 1965.
[19] McDonagh, J. E. R., *The Nature of Disease Up-To-Date*, Heinemann, London, 1946.
[20] Howard, A. E., *Farming and Gardening for Health or Disease*, Faber & Faber, London, 1945.
[21] Voisin, A., *Soil, Grass, and Cancer*, Crosby Lockwood & Son, London, 1959.
[22] Voisin, A., *ibid*, p.191.
[23] Quick, C., 'Some Clinical Aspects of Vegetarian Nutrition', *Brit. Nat. J.* 5:6, 1962, p.173.
[24] Williamson, J., Diet Therapy in Rheumatic Ailments, *Brit. Nat. J.* 7:9, 1967, p.283.
[25] Pfeiffer, C. C., *Mental and Elemental Nutrients*, Keates Publishing Inc., New Canaan, Connecticut, 1975, p.102.
[26] Dummer, T. G., 'Some Negative Experiences with Vegetarianism', *Brit. Nat. J.* 9:4, 1971, p.87.
[27] Weiss, E., Personal communication, April 1982.
[28] Last, W., 'Dangerous Dairy Products', *Brit. Nat. J.* 9:12, Spring 1976, p.312.
[29] Budd, M. L., *Low Blood Sugar*, Thorsons Publishers, Wellingborough, 1981.

[30] Gansslen, quoted in Bircher-Benner, *ibid.*
[31] Bircher-Benner, M., *ibid*, p.91.
[32] Pauling, L., *The Common Cold and Flu*, W. H. Freeman & Co., 1976.
[33] Shute, W. E. and Taub, H., *Vitamin E for Ailing and Healthy Hearts*, W. H. Allen, New York, 1971.
[34] Urbach, E., *Skin Diseases, Nutrition, and Metabolism*, Heinemann, London, 1946.
[35] Shelton, H. M., *The Hygienic System*, Volume III, Shelton's Health School, San Antonio, Texas, 1950, p.101.
[36] Nikolayev, Y. S., *Controlled Fasting Cure of Schizophrenia*, Moscow, 1963.
[37] Sugarman, L., 'Physiological Changes During Fasting II'. *Brit. Nat. J.* 9:9, 1975, p.228.
[38] Sugarman, L., 'Physiological Changes During Fasting III', *Brit. Nat. J.* 9:11, 1975, p.284.
[39] Sugarman, L., *ibid*, p.286.
[40] Moyle, A., 'The Guelpa Fast', *Brit. Nat. J.* 7:10, 1969, p.307.
[41] Pitcairn-Knowles, A., *History and Development of the Schroth Cure*, Riposo, Hastings.
[42] Goodman, J., 'The Hay Diet', *Visual Encyclopaedia of Unconventional Medicine*, Trewin-Copplestone, London, 1978, p.140.
[43] Ellis, F. R., 'Some Hazards Connected with the Use of Animal Milk', *Brit. Nat. J.* 9:7, 1974, p.181.
[44] Denman, A. M., 'Principles of Clinical Immunology', *The Practitioner* 226, December 1982, p.1993.
[45] Cavagni, G., 'Atopic Dermatitis Due to Food Allergens', *The Practitioner* 225:1361, 1981, p.1657.
[46] Mackarness, R., *Not All In The Mind*, Pan Books, London, 1976.
[47] Budd, M. L., *ibid.*

6. Structure and Function

The nutrition, innervation, and drainage of each component of the body is essential for its normal healthy function. If the blood and lymph are denied access to the cells and tissues which they bathe, the essential exchange of oxygen, nutrients, and waste products of metabolism cannot take place, the function of the organs they embody is impaired and they become more susceptible to disease.

The naturopath considers functional integrity to be of paramount importance and, in his assessment of a patient's requirements, will place particular emphasis on the role of the postural alignment of the body and any structural deviations from the norm. Restrictions of joint mobility, postural distortions, and muscle spasms are important, not only because of the local discomfort they may cause, but because of their possible reflex effect on other areas of the body.

Even in those disorders commonly regarded as being primarily of a mechanical nature — such as back pain, joint sprains, and muscle injuries, — the naturopath takes a broader view of the factors which may lie behind the immediate symptoms.

Naturopathic Osteopathy

It is widely believed that osteopathy consists primarily of manipulative techniques suitable only for the relief of joint strains and sprains and for the treatment of structural disorders of the spine. It is, however, much broader in its application and the purely mechanical myth is certainly dispelled in Leon Chaitow's book on osteopathy in this series.[1]

The pioneers of osteopathy and chiropractic, another form of manipulative therapy, used their skills to alleviate a wide range of bodily disorders. Andrew Taylor Still, the founder of osteopathy, introduced the Rule of the Artery which emphasized the dependence on musculo-skeletal freedom of adequate blood flow to internal organs. D. D. Palmer, who pioneered chiropractic, emphasized the importance of vertebral alignment to the nerve supply of these same organs.

In osteopathic parlance a 'lesion' is a structural anomaly, most commonly a vertebral displacement, but it may be regarded as any mechanical or functional deviation from the norm, which can be responsible for symptoms. The naturopathic view of structural lesions coincides closely with that of Still's, and, more particularly, with the Total Lesion Concept of H. H. Fryette. He defined the total lesion as a 'composite of all the various separate individual lesions or factors, mechanical or otherwise, which cause, or predispose to cause, disease from which the patient may be suffering at the moment'.[2]

Most naturopaths are also trained as osteopaths and have to deal with a significant number of spinal and allied disorders. In their diagnostic assessment they will, however, consider more fully the nutritional and emotional influence on a joint problem. Musculo-skeletal disorders are, therefore, viewed not simply as mechanical problems but in terms of the disturbances of the dynamics of body movement.

The popular view of osteopathy is that it is concerned with adjusting displaced vertebrae or relieving 'trapped nerves' by simple manipulation. Whilst this is frequently and effectively the case, the fact that some people regularly have to have 'a bone put back' is indicative of other factors which have not been adequately attended to, such as the balance of muscles and ligaments. It is, in any case, unlikely that change of position occurs after adjustment of most individual vertebrae and it cannot be demonstrated by X-rays before and after treatment. The only positional changes demonstrable are at the pivotal areas of the spinal column, the atlas/axis region, ninth thoracic vertebra, and sacrum.[3] Most vertebral displacements are part of a group lesion in which the osteopathic or chiropractic adjustment effects a release of restricted mobility rather than a significant change of position.

Naturopaths will make such adjustments to bony alignment as are necessary but they will generally be more concerned with the condition of the soft tissues which lie adjacent to the bony lesion, and in particular to the connective tissue.

Collagen

Collagen is the protein-based substance found in the connective tissues of the body. These tissues, of various types, are concerned primarily with supporting body structures and binding parts together. They are also involved in food storage and the body defence mechanisms because, as we saw in Chapter 2, this mesenchymal substance is important as a neutralizer and transporter of endogenous toxins as well as regulating the electrolyte (mineral) balance.

The functional efficiency of connective tissue is, according to Brian K. Youngs, as important as that of any other tissue, and he has pointed out that it has become the 'focal point of manipulative attack for the naturopathic profession'.[4] Appropriately, it was a naturopath who developed a unique form of soft-tissue manipulation, the neuro-muscular technique.

Neuro-muscular Technique

The neuro-muscular technique (NMT) consists of slow, deep, controlled moves by the balls of the thumbs, or palmar surface of the distal phalanges, over connective tissue. It affects the ligaments, aponeuroses, fascial planes, intra-mesenteric, and sub-dermal connective tissues. The movements are, as far as possible, at right angles to the muscle fibres or the white fibres of ligaments and tendons.

The technique was introduced by Stanley Lief, one of the foremost pioneers of natural therapy in the U.K., and bears many similarities to the *Bindegewebmassage,* developed in Germany by Elizabeth Dicke. Its effects are said to be:

decongestion,
restoration of eccentric muscle action and stabilization of articular structures,
increased range of mobility,
reflex effects.[5]

The role of muscles, tendons, and ligaments in structural lesions may be likened to that of the guy-ropes of a tent. The angles and stresses of the vertebrae of the spinal column, and other joints, are affected by the tone of these soft tissues, just as the poles of a tent are dependent on the proper adjustment of the guy-ropes. NMT can, therefore, minimize the amount of manipulation required to articular structures and can be the answer to many of those musculo-skeletal problems which repeatedly have to be manipulated. Leon Chaitow reports excellent results in many acute and chronic structural lesions, where only the gentlest and lightest osteopathic and chiropractic techniques are required when used in conjunction with NMT.[6] It is of particular value where fibrous changes have taken place or where more active procedures would prove painful. NMT is especially adaptable to the frailty of the elderly for whom other manipulative procedures may be contra-indicated.

Abdominal Technique

A special application of the NMT by Lief was his treatment of deep-seated adhesions, contractions, and muscle spasms in the abdominal area. These are particularly prevalent after surgical operations in some patients for whom they can be a source of considerable discomfort. Lief's method of breaking up these aberrant tissue states became known as 'bloodless surgery'.

Chaitow describes them as abdominal release techniques and goes on to say:

> These 'release' techniques can be applied to soft areas of the body (e.g. the throat) as well as to the abdomen. The original concept of 'bloodless surgery' was that adhesions were being 'peeled' away from their anchorage by the technique and in some cases this might have been so. However, its application is to any area of tight, fibrosed, spastic, contracted or adhering soft tissue in the abdominal region. The most dramatic improvements in function are noted after its use in such conditions as spastic or atonic constipation, visceroptosis, dysmenorrhoea, and menorrhagia, as well as ill-defined abdominal congestion and pain.
>
> Precisely what takes place after release technique is open to conjecture. An improvement in tone and circulation, and usually of general function, is the most obvious result. It is a matter of debate whether this is because of a release of a long-held contractive

state in the soft tissues or because of an actual breaking of adhesions or because of some other mechanism.[6]

Lief applied his technique for the release of post-operative adhesions under subdued red light to induce as deep a relaxation as possible.

Nutrition in Structural Disorders

The role of nutrition in the health and defence of the body was considered in the last chapter but it has been difficult to establish a direct correlation between dietary excess or deficiency and musculo-skeletal problems, in spite of the long held naturopathic contention that many collagen diseases, such as rheumatoid arthritis, have a nutritional basis. Modern research does, however, point increasingly to the protective effects of such nutrients as vitamin C on articular surfaces and connective tissues in general.

Naturopaths consider the connective tissue to be particularly important to the integrity of the spine. In some cases of chronic back pain the appearance of the Black Line Phenomenon has suggested an underlying nutritional deficiency.[7] It is a common observation of osteopaths who use a spinal meter, to detect the most active lesions, that pressure on either side of the spine with the hemispherical probe of approximately 0.5cm diameter, will, in some patients, illicit a dark blue or black line. The pressure of the probe is usually very light since it is intended to register variations in skin resistance, but it has a pinching-off effect on the arterioles and venules of the capillary network beneath the skin. Local engorgement of the capillary bed with deoxygenated venous blood causes the appearance of the line which slowly fades as the circulation returns.

Keith Lamont, who first drew attention to the Black Line Phenomenon, has found that administration of vitamin E, bioflavonoid complex (vitamin C + P), and homoeopathic *Ferrum phosphate*, will correct this deficiency.[7] Preliminary data collected by Lamont regarding a possible co-existing blood anomaly showed either low haemoglobin or low serum iron levels, but clearly, more studies are required of this and other nutritional aspects of musculo-skeletal disorders to establish the most effective dietary régime for patients subject to such conditions.

Neurolymphatic Reflexes

In their search for the underlying cause of disorders, naturopaths make frequent recourse to the systems of reflex therapy, such as Chapman's Reflexes. Chapman's Reflexes are palpable gangliform contractions located in specific anatomical areas which can be related to disturbances of specific viscera, or glands *(Figure 10).* These contractions are particularly noticeable in the intercostal spaces of the anterior rib cage, abdominal fasciae, and paravertebral regions, where they may be sought with the palpating finger. The NMT, or inhibitory pressure, will slowly remove them. If a contraction has been present for some time, however, it may have established a very firm reflex influence with a number of secondary trigger points in seemingly unrelated tissues.

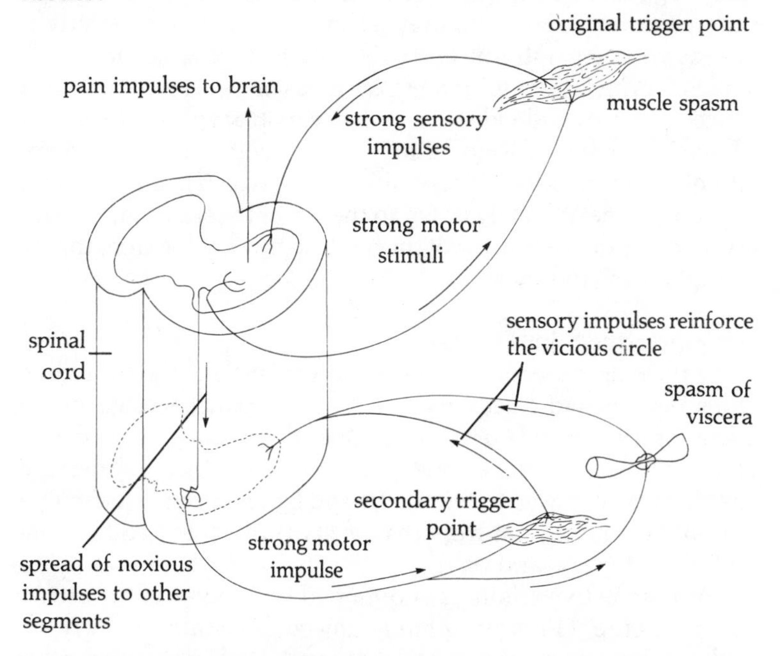

Figure 10. A simplified scheme of the Reflex Arc. Pain impulses from a primary trigger point (e.g. muscle spasm) may be referred to other segments of the spinal cord. These noxious impulses are transmitted by motor nerves to other muscle fibres and visceral structures, such as the intestines, where they cause referred pain. This may persist until the original trigger point is sought and treated.

There is, in neurology, a Law of Facilitation which states that when an impulse passes through a set of neurones it will take the same course on future occasions, thereby reducing the resistance in that route. Faulty postural habits may, therefore, bring back muscle contractions which have been removed, and re-establish a similar pain pattern. Secondary trigger points arise because there is the tendency for a noxious stimulus to spread to other nerve segments and cause contraction at the muscle end-plates of nerves arising from them.[8]

The non-specificity of this approach again emphasizes the naturopathic concern for individuality. There can be no standardized treatment, hence the difficulty in carrying out objective research. Chaitow has said that the treatment becomes the diagnosis.[6] Variations in the anatomy of the nervous system can be quite diverse and may account for differing sensitivity to environmental stimuli and pain arising in seemingly unrelated areas.[9] Whilst fascilitation makes areas of pain reference fairly consistent in the individual, they may vary from person to person. Travell and Biglow found that in twenty eight subjects a trigger point in the sternocleidomastoid muscle, which passes from the mastoid bone obliquely down to the top of the sternum, referred pain to five different areas of the face and head — the chin, throat, temple, ear, and mastoid.[10]

Degenerative Joint Disease

Arthrosis, or degeneration of the joints, such as the shoulders, hips, spine, and knees represents an advanced stage in the deterioration of collagen tissues. Once this damage has occurred there is little that can be done to reverse it, but, by the systematic application of NMT to tendinous and ligamentous attachments around the joints, naturopaths are generally able to offer some relief of stiffness and pain.

A more active stimulus is obtained by the use of an extract of mistletoe *(Viscum album)* injected intramuscularly or subcutaneously in wheals around the affected joint, or on either side of the affected vertebral segment. The strength of the extract is increased serially and injections must be given at not more than seven-day intervals until the required strength is reached. *Viscum album* evokes inflammatory changes which reactivate fibrous tissue and restore some elasticity to the collagen.

In one study of 253 cases of arthrosis deformans of the knee joint, treated by injections of *Viscum album* in Germany, 87.7 per cent showed a beneficial response with both relief of pain and restoration of mobility.[11] In another study of 247 cases of osteo-arthrosis of the spine with disc degeneration, 131 became symptom-free, 81 improved, and 25 were unaffected.[12]

The Mind and Muscles

The influence of the emotions on physical health has been well established in the field of psychosomatic medicine. The dynamics of this relationship are well described by Franz Alexander:

> In the little child the most primitive expression of frustration is random motor discharge. If, through punitive measures, this discharge becomes associated with fear and guilt, then in later life whenever fear and guilt arise there results a psychological 'strait jacket'. These patients try to achieve an equilibrium between aggressive impulses and control. They learn to discharge aggression through muscular activity in acceptable channels: hard work, sports, gardening, actively heading the house. They also learn to relieve the restrictive influence of the conscience by serving others. Whenever this equilibrium is disturbed by specific events which interrupt the adaptive mode of discharging hostility and relieving guilt the chronic inhibited aggression leads to increased muscle tonus and in some way to arthritis . . . [13]

The psychiatrist Wilhelm Reich was one of the first to explain more fully the way in which unresolved emotional conflicts could give rise to restrictions of mobility in areas such as the neck and shoulders.[14]

Naturopaths make use of soft tissue procedures, such as NMT, to release the physical tensions related to emotional conflicts — an approach to psychological disorders pioneered by Reich. The full expression of blocked emotions is often essential before some musculo-skeletal problems can be resolved.

Postural Re-education

To achieve any lasting improvement of musculo-skeletal disorders, the patient needs to develop an awareness of bodily tensions and the faulty patterns of use which may have given rise to them. Naturopaths generally endeavour to educate the patient in correct use of the body according to the principles of F. Matthias Alexander.[15] Alexander discovered, by personal experience with throat problems, how faulty postural habit patterns could interfere with proper circulation and drainage and he evolved a system of postural re-education which develops an awareness of the gravitational forces acting on the body, and its use in such a way as to minimize the stress on joints and ligaments. This integrates well with the holistic naturopathic approach to musculo-skeletal dynamics.

Exercise

The role of the patient in the techniques described so far in this chapter may appear to be a rather passive one. In practice, however, the patient's personal responsibility for postural awareness, exercise, and, when indicated, rest, is strongly emphasized. During episodes of acute pain, rest is essential in a position which will minimize the strain on affected joints. For back pain this will generally mean lying flat on a firm but comfortable surface, such as a mattress on the floor.

Where back problems are associated with vertebral misalignment naturopaths are opposed to the use of exercise as a form of treatment without osteopathic guidance. They point out that stretching and bending exercises may merely loosen already hypermobile joints while areas of hypomobility may become more fixed. Once spinal alignment has been corrected osteopathically exercise systems, such as yoga or Tai Chi, are recommended as ways of maintaining mobility and spinal tone.

Naturopaths recommend any form of regular exercise which is enjoyable, uses a wide range of muscles and joints, and makes the lungs work to their fullest capacity. Members of the British Naturopathic and Osteopathic Association have, however, expressed concern about fitness and aerobics classes run by people with insufficient experience to discriminate between the various capabilities of their pupils. Vigorous jerking movements can be hazardous to those who are susceptible to back injuries.

REFERENCES

[1] Chaitow, L., *Osteopathy — A Complete Health Care System,*

Thorsons Publishers, Wellingborough, 1982.
[2] Fryette, H. H., *Principles of Osteopathic Technique*, Academy of Applied Osteopathy, Carmel, California, 1954.
[3] Bradbury, P., *The Mechanics of Healing*, Peter Owen, London, 1967.
[4] Youngs, B. K., 'Some Aspects of Connective Tissue', *Brit. Nat. J.* 5:4, 1962, p.116.
[5] Youngs, B. K., 'Physiological Background of Neuromuscular Technique', *Brit. Nat. J.* 5:6, 1962, p.176.
[6] Chaitow, L., *Neuro-muscular Technique*, Thorsons Publishers, Wellingborough, 1980.
[7] Lamont, K., 'Black Line Phenomenon — Regional Capillary Anoxia', *Brit. Nat. J.* 9:3, 1970.
[8] Vannerson, J. F. and Nimmo, R. L., 'Specificity and the Law of Fascilitation in the Nervous System', *The Receptor* 2:1, Granbury, Texas, 1971.
[9] Williams, R., *Biochemical Individuality*, University of Texas Press, Austin, Texas, 1956.
[10] Travell, J. and Biglow, N. H., 'Role of Somatic Trigger Areas in the Patterns of Hysteria', *Psychosomatic Medicine* 9:6, 1947.
[11] Fischer, J. and Lussenhop, H., 'Zur Therapie der Arthrosis Deformans des Kniegelenkes', *Ärztliche Praxis* 4:2, 1952.
[12] Foulkes, G. L., 'Viscum Album and its use in Osteoarthritic, Fibrotic, and Carcinomatous Conditions', *J. Res. Soc. Nat. Thera.*, Spring 1977.
[13] Alexander, F., *Psychosomatic Medicine*, Allen & Unwin, London, 1952, p.205.
[14] Reich, W., *Character Analysis*, Vision Press, London, 1950.
[15] Alexander, F. M., *Use of the Self*, Integral Press, Bexley, 1946.

7. Natural Stimuli — Water, Air and Sunlight

The skin is a very important organ. It is the mediator between the body and its environment and is well adapted to this role by its functions as a sense organ, insulator, protector, and eliminator. It is richly supplied with nerve endings, especially on the hands and feet, which can detect the subtlest changes of texture and form. It has blood vessels which regulate heat loss and fatty tissues which insulate. It has elastic tissues and cell layers which give resilience and maintain a defence against invading organisms, and it has pores which can excrete fluids containing waste matter, as well as cells which can take up and absorb other substances from its surroundings. Not surprisingly, the skin plays a major role in naturopathic therapy.

The eliminative functions of the skin are considered to be a vital supplement to those of the bowels, lungs, and kidneys. It gives off 500-900ml of sweat per day which may contain over 10g of solids and is, therefore, referred to by some authorities as the 'third kidney'. The male has more sweat glands than the female (who eliminates toxins with the menses) so skin function assumes even greater importance to long-term health in the male.[1]

The suppression of skin rashes and discharges depresses the eliminative functions of the skin and gives rise to the exudative diathesis which carries a susceptibility to respiratory or rheumatic disorders.

Another valuable attribute of the skin is its reflex connections with other vital organs. Stimuli can be applied to the skin to regulate the functions of the heart, lungs, stomach, liver, spleen, and kidneys, as well as the circulation to those areas. The primary effect of any stimulus to the skin leads to a secondary effect which may, in turn, benefit the whole organism. The reflex benefits of skin stimuli on the lungs will lead in turn to a constitutional improvement.

The stimuli which are applied are those to which, in natural circumstances, the skin would normally be exposed, but which in the modern environment it rarely meets in an effective form. They are air, sunlight, and water. The most extensively used and systematized as a therapy is water.

HYDROTHERAPY

The use of water as a physical stimulus goes back to very early times. The properties imparted to water by certain geological features were well known to the Romans who established spas, which still operate, at such sites in different parts of Europe. The systematic application of water as a therapeutic agent did not take place until the nineteenth century when American and European scientists, most notably a Bavarian priest, Father Sebastian Kneipp, classified the uses of water as a therapeutic stimulus. His book, *My Water Cure,* is regarded as one of the classics of hydrotherapy and throughout Germany today there are many centres devoted to the practice of *Kneipptherapie.*

Water possesses several properties which make it an excellent therapeutic agent.[2]

Power of absorbing heat
Solvent properties
Ease of transformation to solid, liquid, or gaseous form

Water can, therefore, be used as a medium for the administration of medicinal substances and nutrients but it is its thermo-regulatory effects which form the basis of its application in hydrotherapy as an alternative to other stimuli, such as dry heat.

There are two major categories of hydrotherapy, external applications, such as baths, sprays, and compresses, and internal applications, such as inhalations and enemas.

External Hydrotherapy

The skin has two main types of nerve endings which are concerned with temperature regulation, the warm receptors, which regulate the maximum heat tolerance of the skin, and the cold receptors which respond to cold stimuli.[3]

There are also reflex connections of the skin's surface with internal organs in a segmental pattern, known as Heads Zones. These are based on the distribution of cutaneous nerve branches from the spinal cord which have a common route with deeper branches to the respective organs. By virtue of this common origin, areas supplied by the superficial branch of a nerve are in reflex connection with the organs supplied by the deeper branch. These reflex areas are used extensively in hydrotherapy as well as diagnostically. There are several possible routes of influence established by these nerve pathways:

viscero-visceral reflex (from one organ to another)
viscero-cutaneous reflex (from an organ to the skin)
viscero-motor reflex (from organ to activating nerve)
cutaneo-visceral reflex (from skin to organ)

As we saw in Chapter 5, noxious stimuli in one area are capable of eliciting a trophic response in another, and this same mechanism can be turned to therapeutic advantage.

Effects of Cold Applications

The application of cold water to the body elicits a *primary effect* of vital depression with constriction of blood vessels. This is utilized to regulate vital activity in the treatment of surface pain and inflammation. If the cold application is brief, there is a *secondary effect* in which pallor gives way to dilatation of the fine capillaries and arterioles in the skin. There is, therefore, an increased rate of circulatory exchange, the blood conveying inflammatory waste products away from, and oxygen and vital substances to the injured area more effectively.

Local cold applications in the form of sprays or packs are also known to have *reflex effects* due to stimulation of sympathetic nerve ganglia in the vessel walls. For example, cold applications to the lower one third of the sternum stimulate renal function and a prolonged cold footbath causes contraction of the vessels of the uterus which may be of value in counteracting uterine haemorrhage.[4] Cold applications will also stimulate activity of muscles owing to the promotion of their nutrition. Hydrotherapy is, therefore, extensively used in the treatment of atrophic and spastic paralyses.[5]

The indiscriminate use of reflex stimulation is not without its hazards, as Thomson points out that it may encourage the development of a local fontanelle for the discharge of poisonous matter.[6] In naturopathic practice care is always taken to ensure that general eliminative functions are sustained to prevent overloading an unnatural channel of discharge.

Effects of Hot Applications

Hot applications have a *primary effect* of excitation to the brain and nervous system whereas the *secondary effect* is depressant through reflex action. Prolonged application of heat increases heat production and may lead to eventual exhaustion, either locally, in specific organs deprived of blood drawn to the surface, or generally. The enervating effect of prolonged hot baths is a well-known example.

There are, however, certain physiological benefits of hot applications. Unless followed by cold, for example, hot applications increase the white blood cell count and decrease the red cells. Prolonged hot applications over abdominal areas increase the secretions of the stomach and liver. Some of the general benefits of raised body temperature are summarized as follows:

anti-bacterial effect
anti-viral effect — inhibition of non-specific virus multiplication
— promotion of interferon synthesis
cytostatic effect
increased leukocytosis
regulation of phagocytosis
antiphlogistic effect
stimulation of immune reaction
promotion of effects of medicinal substances[7]

The deliberate elevation of body temperature, known as fever therapy, to achieve some of these effects has already been referred to in Chapter 4.

Alternate Hot and Cold Applications

Contrast bathing is commonly recommended in naturopathic practice. A short hot application followed by a shorter or equal cold application is excitant in effect. The heat is sufficient to cause excitation of circulation and vital function which is neutralized by the cold application leading to a constriction of blood vessels. The skin is then prepared for a new excitant effect, the overall result being one of excitation with increased circulatory exchange.[8]

Methods of Application

There are many ways of applying hydrotherapy externally, such as baths, sprays, and compresses, the choice being made primarily on the basis of the patient's constitution as well as the facilities available in the home. Residential naturopathic clinics are usually equipped with sitz baths and other hydrotherapy units, but the patient being treated from an office practice can generally devise effective stimuli with hot and cold water and some towels or sheets. The constitution of the patient dictates the choice and intensity of the stimulus. Sudden contrasts of temperature or wide application of extreme stimuli, such as sprays and baths, would not be well tolerated by the very young or the frail and elderly.

Washing, Sprays, and Baths

The most common and convenient way of applying water therapeutically is by immersion. The whole body, up to the neck, or part of it such as the arms, legs, or lower torso, are immersed in water of an appropriate temperature, either hot or alternating with cold.

Full baths are often used not only as a physical stimulus but to apply substances with therapeutic properties such as mineral or herbal agents. Epsom salts (magnesium sulphate) or sodium bicarbonate are often added for their diaphoretic (sweat inducing) and alkaline properties. Many herbal agents may be used, such as hay-flowers or oat-straw, the latter recommended by Kneipp for complaints of the kidneys and bladder.[9] The ingredients are usually boiled and the decoction is added to the bath.

Another ingredient, extensively used in Europe, is the Moor Bath, which contains a peat extract. Moor baths have a wide range of indications and in the gynaecological field alone H. Baatz states that they are of value in chronic inflammatory conditions of the genital area, vegetative and generative ovarian deficiency, sterility, habitual abortion, arrested genital development in puberty, dysmenorrhoea, senile atrophy, pruritis vulvae, and post-operative complications, among others.[10] Moor baths are said to work by stimulation of the circulation of the splanchnic and hypogastric areas (abdominal areas), as well as by percutaneous absorption of oestrogenic substances. Various clinics specializing in the treatment of gynaecological disorders have achieved an overall success rate of 47.5 per cent in the treatment of sterility due to ovarian insufficiency.[10]

Moor baths have been particularly noted for their benefits in the treatment of rheumatic disorders. Hyaluronidase is an enzyme found in body tissues which increases the permeability of connective tissue and leads to a destruction of the joint surfaces in degenerative joint disease, such as arthritis. A distinct reduction in hyaluronidase activity was noted after a series of moor bath treatments.[11] It is likely that there is also some restoration of the elasticity of tendons and ligaments with such treatment but this is not easy to assess objectively.

Local baths include *sitz baths*, which are generally given in pairs. The patient sits immersed to the waist in hot or cold water whilst his feet are placed in water of a contrasting temperature. Alternate hot and cold sitz baths are given as both a general tonic and a stimulus to the abdominal and pelvic areas and are a valuable adjunctive treatment for conditions in which stasis or prolapse is a common feature, such as diverticulosis, haemorrhoids, and gynaecological problems. For most contrast baths the temperature of the warm water should be about 38°C (100°F) and the cold 16-22°C (60-72°F).[12]

Other local reflex areas such as the arms or feet are bathed in either hot and cold, or cold water only. Immersion of the extremities in cold water for short periods before retiring is said to be conducive to good sleep. A feature of Kneipptherapie clinics in Germany are special tanks containing water at 10-18°C (50-65°F), through which patients may wade barefoot before retiring.

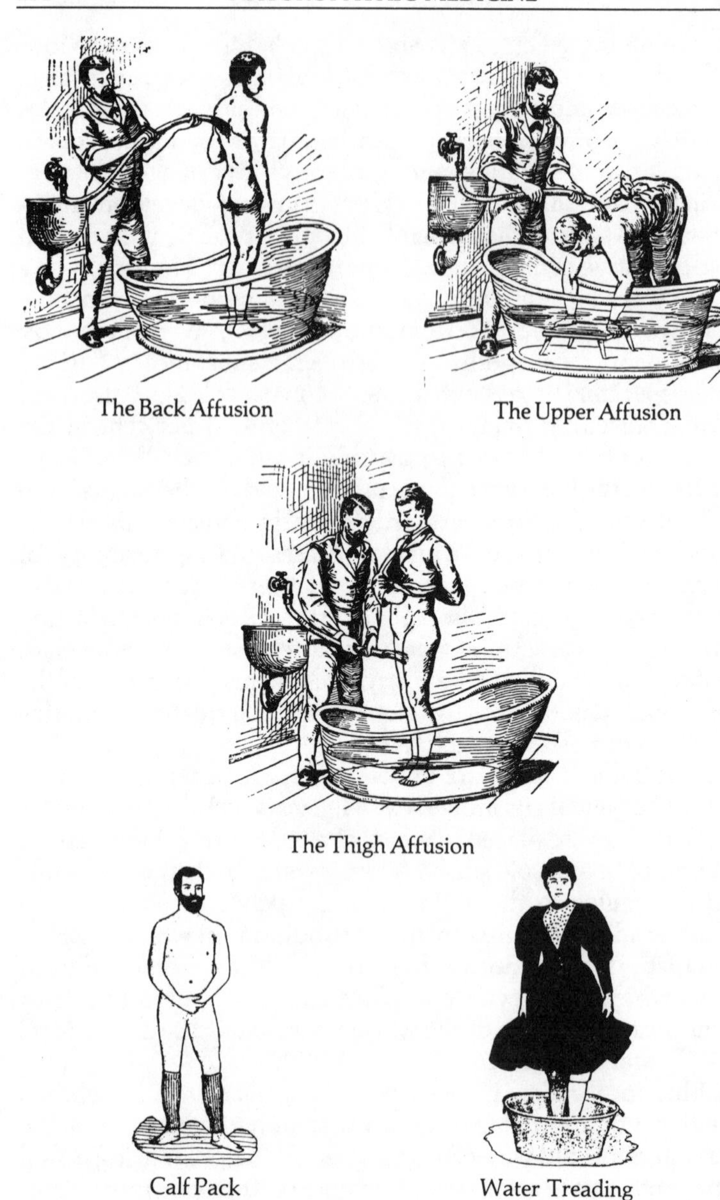

The Back Affusion

The Upper Affusion

The Thigh Affusion

Calf Pack

Water Treading

Figure 11. Hydrotherapy illustrations from a nineteenth century health manual (*The Natural Method of Healing* by F. E. Bilz, 1898).

Water *spraying* is a way of localizing the hot or cold stimulus to the muscular reflex areas. A water hose, preferably with a strong jet, is directed at the skin and moved to and fro in a systematic fashion *(Figure 11)*. In the treatment of the knee or shoulder, for example, Bruggemann recommends directing the jet to different areas of the skin over the joints for periods of five seconds.[12] The duration of the applications to the whole area will be adjusted according to the constitution of the patient. Strong cold jets applied to spinal areas provide a particularly strong tonic to the sympathetic nervous system.

Fomentations, Compresses, and Packs

Stimuli are often applied to the skin with cloths soaked in water of an appropriate temperature. Cotton, flannelette, or towelling, are most suitable. After soaking, the material is wrung out and applied direct to the surface of an area such as a joint, or to the whole body.

Fomentations are generally applied for short duration and will usually be hot, or contrasting hot and cold. The hot applications will be for three to four minutes immediately followed by a cold one for one minute. They may be applied alternately for periods of up to thirty minutes depending upon the severity of the condition and the vital reserve of the patient. Towelling is the most suitable material. Hot fomentations are used in cases of internal congestion, or spasm, such as acute asthmatic paroxyms, where the dilatation of surface blood vessels, induced by the heat, affords some relief of the deeper congestion. Contrasting fomentations are widely used in naturopathic practice as a stimulus to circulatory and lymphatic drainage in a variety of conditions. They are of value in many long-standing disorders where tonic effects are required, for example, in chronic bronchitis, or emphysema, and are of particular benefit in acute painful episodes, such as low back pain, where heat alone would be liable to aggravate inflammatory processes.

Compresses are used also for localized application, but usually of longer duration. Flannelette or cotton material is soaked in cold water and applied damp to a joint or reflex area. It may then be covered with an outer wrap of thicker material which can partially retain the heat which is generated as a reaction to the initial cold stimulus. Cold compresses are generally applied to swollen and painful joints, sprains, and areas of inflammation. They are most suitable for the smaller joints, such as knees, wrists, and ankles, or for areas such as the throat.

Packs may take many forms but are usually designed to cover larger areas. The *whole body pack* or Scottish mantle, consists of a wet sheet which is wrapped around the body from the neck downwards. A *trunk pack* is wrapped around the body from the armpit to groin and an *abdominal pack* from the waist to the groin. In each case the inner wrap is soaked in cold water and, after application, one or more layers of towelling or blanket are wrapped around to retain the heat generated. The patient may lie in the pack for several hours. Hot water bottles are usually placed at the feet, and cold compresses may also be applied to the throat or head in cases of fever.

Body packs are indicated in many chronic disorders where a stimulation of the eliminative functions of the skin is desired. In naturopathic practice packs are most commonly used in the treatment of febrile diseases, particularly in children. The thermoregulatory effect of the pack serves to induce a perspiration which relieves internal heat. Cold packs are a relatively strong stimulus which would be contra-indicated for the very young, the elderly, and those of delicate constitution.

Steam Applications

Heat applied by means of steam is a general stimulus to the eliminative functions of the skin. Saunas or steam cabinets are used to raise the body temperature and induce perspiration. The treatment is generally concluded with a cold shower or plunge to equalize the circulation.

Cryotherapy

The use of ice as a cold stimulus is considered unsuitable except in extreme circumstances, such as severe inflammation or pain. Direct use of ice on the skin is liable to be damaging to the cells. Ice can, however, be used to cool the water for cold compresses.

Poultices

Although not strictly classified under hydrotherapy, poultices are an external application commonly used in naturopathic practice. The analgesic properties of heat are combined with the therapeutic benefits of medicinal plants or mineral substances. The vegetable matter is generally placed in a bag of a porous material which may then be heated before application.

The *hay-flower* pack consists of a selection of spring herbs in a porous bag, which has been steeped in hot water for five to ten minutes before being applied to the neck and shoulder area. This is said to be of value for cases of insomnia and nervous tension.[13]

A *cabbage poultice* is one of a variety of vegetable applications. Macerated or chopped cabbage leaves are applied to swellings, particularly the effusions of joints afflicted, for example, with rheumatoid arthritis.

Internal Hydrotherapy

Several types of internal hydrotherapeutic application are made in naturopathic practice.

Enemas have long been a part of the natural therapy régime. Water, usually at body temperature, but sometimes cooler, is injected into the rectum by means of a catheter attached to a tube leading from the container. The water is retained for five to ten minutes before evacuation. This cleanses the lower bowel of faecal matter, some of which, it is believed, may have lodged in the folds of the rectum and been bypassed by normal faecal transit.

Enemas are considered to be a valuable adjunct to fasting and other cleansing régimes. Apart from their cleansing function the gradual injection of cooler water, starting at body temperature and reducing in sequence of injections to 15°C (60°F), can be of benefit in febrile conditions. The enema enjoys much less popularity with modern naturopaths, who consider it may interfere with natural intestinal secretions and the bacterial flora. Enemas are, in any case, only suitable for patients who have been fasting for at least twenty-four hours and in whom most normal faecal waste will have been eliminated.

Colonic Irrigations

Colonic irrigations are used in many residential naturopathic clinics for patients who have been fasting or on a light diet for several days. The apparatus permits injection of water at body temperature which then flows out by means of a two-way tube, the process being repeated for 30-40 minutes. This helps to loosen adherent faecal matter.

The colonic irrigation, valued by some practitioners as an adjunct to the treatment of chronic catarrhal disorders and skin problems, is opposed by some naturopaths because, like the enema, it may disturb the normal secretions of the colon and the essential bacterial colonies which they harbour.

Inhalation

The respiratory membranes are an active and receptive surface and, like the intestines, have the same primary cellular structure as the skin. Inhalation of steam is often used to stimulate the mucous membranes of nose and sinuses and to mobilize catarrhal secretions. Various herbal extracts or aromatic oils may be added to the water to increase the stimulus. The most famous of these, Friars Balsam, is a resinoid of the plant, which loosens bronchial secretions. Some naturopaths consider this to be too irritant to mucous membranes and, therefore, not an acceptable treatment.

AIR

Air of sufficient purity is, of course, important for oxygenation via the lungs but it also has properties which make it a valuable stimulus to the skin. McKie lists the following reasons for its value as a thermal agent:

absorbs heat
circulates around body
continuous contact with skin
variable temperature
absorbs moisture from body surface.[14]

There may also be antiseptic properties and the Continental practice of hanging bedding from the window to air is not entirely without reason.

Air baths are recommended by practitioners for their general tonic effects and promotion of non-specific resistance. Because it forms part of a more general therapeutic régime there is little objective evidence of the benefits of air baths but they are considered to be most effective for respiratory conditions. It is an old medical practice to place TB sufferers in the open air for long periods of convalescence. Exercise increases the respiratory exchange and maintains the temperature of the body whilst it is exposed to air.

Ionization

Some of the benefits of air in mountainous regions (where TB sanataria are often located), near waterfalls, and in the countryside generally, may be attributed to its higher content of negative ions. The molecules of oxygen, nitrogen, and carbon dioxide in air can lose electrons for various reasons, particularly around buildings or in polluted atmospheres, and they become positively charged. If they gain electrons they become negatively charged. These charged molecules are called positive or negative ions respectively. The air in mountainous areas, the open country, and after thunderstorms, is richly ionized — that is, it has a high proportion of negative ions. Experimental evidence has shown that higher mammals, including man, thrive in a negatively-charged atmosphere.

Negative ions can be produced electronically in equipment using a high voltage technique which acts rather like a lightning flash. Such ionizers are used in surgeries and offices to create a healthier working environment and therapeutically they have been found to be of value when used regularly by sufferers from a variety of disorders, particularly those in the respiratory field such as rhinitis, sinusitis, hay-fever, asthma, and other allergies.[15]

Although ionization constitutes a non-specific stimulus in the naturopathic sense, research into its uses is still at a comparatively early stage. Some of the physiological effects which have been established are:

increase in vital capacity
increased ciliary activity in the membranes of the lungs
reduction of heart rate and blood-pressure
inhibition of serotonin
reduction of histamine output
normalization of endocrine functions

Some of these effects may be accounted for by the serotin-reducing effect of negative ions. Serotin, or 5-hydroxytryptamine (5HT), is a widely distributed neuro-hormone which plays an important part in the transmission of nerve impulses as well as many other metabolic processes. Significant physiological changes in the endocrine glands and the central nervous system were observed experimentally as a result of air ion exposure to rats and mice.[16]

In order to eliminate the effect of the psychological factor, likely in older children and adults with asthma, Dr Yoram Palti and his colleages at Bikur Holin Hospital, Hadassah Medical School, Jerusalem, conducted a trial of the use of negative ions for the treatment of nineteen infants under one year old. All the children with a diagnosis of asthmatic bronchitis were placed in an atmosphere enriched with negative ions. As a control they were matched with nineteen infants admitted to another hospital with the same diagnosis but who were treated by conventional methods. It was found that negative ions, without any supportive treatment (including antibiotics) terminated attacks of respiratory spasm after a much shorter period than that required by conventional modes of treatment. There was a rebound spasm on withdrawal from the ionized atmosphere but this was not severe and after a short additional period of exposure the infants required no further treatment.[17]

SUNLIGHT

The suns rays provide a radiant heat stimulus which causes burning of various degrees. Its deeper action causes dilatation of blood vessels which relieves congestion internally. The protective pigmentation of the skin leads to tanning and, although suntan induces a sense of well-being, there is no objective evidence that it is beneficial to health.

Artificial radiant heat penetrates the tissues more effectively than conductive heat and, where the heat producing ability of the body is poor, the radiant heat is the preferable stimulus. Both forms, however, are used in naturopathic establishments to induce sweating and are better endured by patients than any other form of sudorific treatment. Radiant heat is said to be of benefit for anaemia, rheumatic disorders, neuralgia, and neurasthenia.[18]

Colour

Within the visible light spectrum individual colours are believed to have a therapeutic influence. The importance of colour selection in interior design is being increasingly recognized, and many dentists, for example, have a blue décor in their waiting rooms and surgeries because of the calming effect this is said to have. Blue colours lower the pulse rate and increase the depth of respiration and are, therefore, beneficial to asthmatics.[19]

Some naturopaths apply the colour principle therapeutically by exposing patients to light filtered with the appropriate colour. Blue light, as already indicated, may be used to induce a state of calm and improve exhalation. Red light, on the contrary, is more stimulating, raises the pulse rate and encourages physical activity.[20]

Full Spectrum Light

Although exposure to a narrow range of the spectrum for short periods appears to have specific benefits, some people are disturbed by long exposure to artificial light, especially fluorescent tubes, which have a shorter wavelength than natural daylight. Children in classrooms under cool white light from conventional fluorescent tubes showed signs of hyperactivity but became calmer when full spectrum lighting was provided. Full spectrum lighting has a longer wavelength more closely resembling that of natural daylight.

Calcium absorption has also been found to be better in individuals exposed to full spectrum light than those under cool white fluorescent tubes.[21] In another investigation it was found that the serum bilirubin levels of premature infants suffering from jaundice were lowered after exposure to sunlight.[22] The infants' eyes were masked during treatment with sunlight so it appears that the skin was the receptor, but many observations have suggested that the eyes are important as receptors of full spectrum light. Its beneficial effects are believed to be meditated through the pituitary gland which receives light stimuli via the optic chiasma.[21] For this reason many naturopaths do not advocate prolonged wearing of sunglasses but encourage instead adequate exposure to natural light, not only for the body as a whole, but in particular for the eyes so that the normal accommodation mechanisms may be made to function fully.

REFERENCES

[1] Issels, J., *Cancer — A Second Opinion*, Hodder and Stoughton, London, 1975, p.70.
[2] McKie, W. L., *Scientific Hydrotherapy*, Health Research, Mokelumne Hill, California, 1957.
[3] Muller-Limmroth, W., 'Neurophysiologische Grundlagen der Kneipptherapie', *Kneipptherapie*, Springer-Verlag, Heidelberg, 1980.
[4] McKie, W. L., *ibid*, p.20.
[5] Rulffs, W., 'Möglichkeiten der Kneipptherapie in der Klinik', *Kneipptherapie, ibid*, p.442.
[6] Thomson, J. C., *Nature Cure from the Inside*, Kingston Clinic, Edinburgh, 1953.
[7] Gehrke, A. and Drexel, H., 'Grundlagen der Bäderbehandlung', *Kneipptherapie, ibid*, p.42.
[8] McKie, W. L., *ibid*, p.31.
[9] Kneipp, S., *My Water Cure*, J. Koesel, Kempten, Bavaria, 1897.
[10] Baatz, H., *Balneotherapie der Frauenkrankheiten*, Deutscher Baderverband eV, Bonn, 1979.
[11] Evers, A., *Balneotherapie degenerativer Erkrankungen der Wirbelsaule*, Deutscher Baderverband eV, Bonn, 1974.
[12] Bruggemann, W., 'Technik der Kneipp Hydrotherapie', *Kneipptherapie, ibid*, p.94.
[13] Bruggemann, W., *ibid*, p.88.
[14] McKie, W. L., *ibid*, p.4.
[15] *A Short How and Why of Air Ionisation*, Leaflet published by Medion, Oxted, Surrey.
[16] Krugger, A. P. and Reed, E. J., 'Biological Impact of Small Air Ions', *Science* 193, September 1976.
[17] Palti, Y., deNour, E. and Abrahamov, A., 'The Effect of Atmospheric Ions on the Respiratory System of Infants', *Pediatrics* 36:3, 1966, pp.405-411.
[18] McKie, W. L., *ibid*.
[19] Gimbel, T., *Healing Through Colour*, C. W. Daniel Co., Saffron Walden, 1980.
[20] Gimbel, T., *ibid*, p.84.
[21] Ott, J. N., *Health and Light*, Pocket Books, New York, 1976.
[22] Cramer, R. J., et al, 'Influence of Light on the Hyperbilirubinaemia in Infants', *The Lancet* 1:1227, 1958.

8. Body, Mind and Spirit

There can be few practitioners of any medical discipline who do not recognize the important therapeutic role of their interaction with the patient. A small amount of time spent on explanation and reassurance in the surgery can significantly improve the ability of the patient to cope with everyday life.[1]

There are very few naturopaths who do not see part of their role of educators in healthy living as being counsellors and providing some guidance to patients on the development of their own resources at every level. Real health means each individual having the capacity to live life to its fullest potential and implies freedom, not only from physical disorders, but also from emotional infirmity. The conflicts arising out of suppressed anger and frustration, or the depression born of repetitive failure and an inability to cope can be as crippling as the most severe physical disorder. In some cases they can also lead to those same physical symptoms. The annals of psychosomatic medicine are heavy with reports of the psychodynamic patterns which have contributed to arthritis, heart disease, respiratory disorders, and many other overtly physical ailments.

Naturopaths try to maintain an awareness of what Lindlahr referred to as 'the three-fold nature of man' when he wrote 'the physical body, with its material elements, is dominated and guided by the mind. The mind is inspired through the inner consciousness which is an attribute of the soul'.[2] To explore this further would be to venture too far into the realms of philosophy for the purpose of this book but suffice it to say that the mind is considered to have a powerful influence over the body, both as a cause of physical illness and a force for healing.

The interpretation of affective (emotion-inducing) processes has made great strides during the twentieth century inspired primarily by the work of Freud, Adler, and Jung. (The acceptance of the principles of Freudian psychoanalysis as a valid hypothesis may have set a precedent for many of the alternative therapies, such as naturopathy, which are also in the frequent position of being unable to meet the rigorous standards of scientific methodology.) While the analytical approach has clearly made the nature of the psychoneuroses more understandable, naturopaths have endeavoured to apply a more unifying concept to the management of emotional disorders — one which has sought to avoid the duality of the body/mind.

In his management of psychoneurosis each practitioner endeavours to establish the connections between the patient's present symptoms and recent events, such as family relationships, as well as past events, such as relationships with parents. Understanding of the psychodynamic patterns created by these inter-relationships is often most enlightening and can prove fruitful at an intellectual level but naturopaths also try to establish the relationships of structural and biochemical factors to the emotions in terms of the triad of basic function (see page 26). This interaction is the basis of psychosomatic medicine which, like naturopathy, has developed more fully during the last sixty years.

Psychosomatic Medicine

Psychological symptoms are based on the activity of the central nervous system which controls our external relationships. Neurovegetative disorders — those organic and functional disturbances which may be attributed to emotional factors — involve a disturbance in the division of labour of the autonomic nervous system. Under conditions of equilibrium the sympathetic nervous system controls our conscious and outwardly directed impulses, such as those concerned with anger or fear. It prepares the body for 'fight or flight' by raising the heart rate, elevating the blood-pressure and blood-sugar level, and increasing the tone of the muscles. The parasympathetic nervous system regulates our internal functions such as digestion, and promotes secretion of digestive juices, contraction of the intestinal tract, and also slows the heart rate. The parasympathetic system is made up by nerves of the cranial and sacral area, of which the tenth cranial nerve, the vagus, exercises the major controlling function over the digestive organs.

The thwarting of these basic survival mechanisms, it is suggested, may explain the physiological processes whereby the inadequate discharge of the expressive emotions can lead to physical illness. Psychosomatic (*psyche*, mind; *soma*, body) medicine is based on the determination of these factors, often subconscious, and therapy is directed to counselling the patient towards an understanding and resolution of their conflict. The physiological processes leading to functional disease were suggested by Franz Alexander.[3]

Repeated conflict, striving, and aggression prepares the body physically to fight or run away. The sympathetic nervous system predominates and if there is little or no discharge of these aggressive impulses physical disorders, such as migraine, arthritis, and heart troubles may develop. Conversely, the desire to withdraw from outwardly directed activity emphasizes a parasympathetic tone, which calls for a fulfilment of infantile dependent needs. Alexander suggests that the frustration of these needs can be causative factors in the onset of neuro-vegetative disorders involving principally those organs under control of the vagus nerve — the stomach (ulcers), lungs (asthma), and intestines (colitis) (see *Figure 12*). In other words, emotions which are repressed and cannot be discharged through the normal channels are converted to physical symptoms which serve partially as a release and partially as a defence against their expression. For many years these theories formed the interpretive basis of naturopathic psychotherapy.

Naturopathic Psychotherapy

In a series of papers in the *British Naturopathic Journal*, and in his book *An Outline of Naturopathic Psychotherapy*, Milton Powell has laid down some of the principles of psychotherapeutic management.[4] These are that:

The patient is not to be regarded as having a mind in a body but

as constituting a mind-body unity.
Mental, emotional, and physical factors act and react upon each other producing either health or disease.
The organism has the power of self-regulation and repair and, if not frustrated through interference, to correct wrong physical habits or bad environment.
Similarly it has the power to maintain mental health, to withstand a varying amount of emotional stress and even to correct or neutralize the wrong mento-emotional habits and bad psychological environment.

It is because man is compelled to live in an imperfectly evolved social environment, Powell suggests, and has not yet mastered the use of the mind-body organism, that physical and mental ill-health are so widespread. That there are many obstacles to emotional self-regulation in modern life becomes increasingly evident from the enormous consumption of tranquillizers, anti-depressants, and sleeping tablets. 'The function of naturopathic psychotherapy is to discover those impediments and so far as man's own personal mistakes are concerned, to provide practical techniques for their removal', Powell wrote. He went on to discuss the scope of naturopathic psychotherapy, maintaining that the

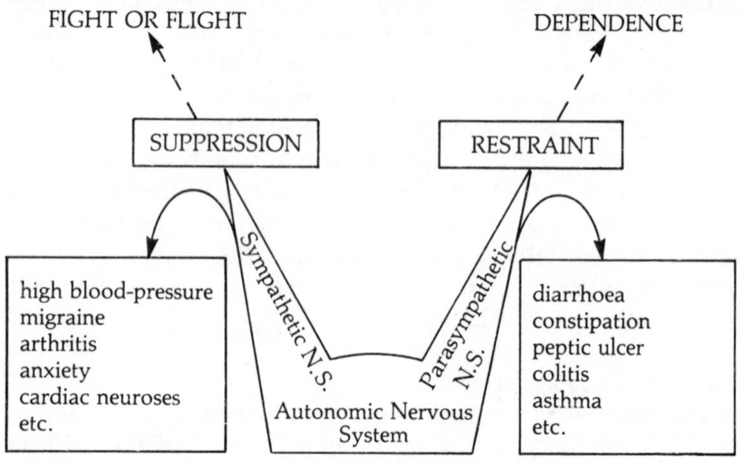

Figure 12. Development of psychosomatic illnesses. The continual blocking of normal hostile tendencies (expressed through the sympathetic nervous system), or the restraint of dependent tendencies (parasympathetic nervous system) may lead to physical disorders.

psychosomatic disorders are the most fruitful field for therapy. Accordingly, naturopaths have evolved an essentially interpretive approach, drawing on a wide field of psychotherapeutic procedures with the use of relaxation techniques as an aid to releasing physical tensions which act as blocks to the free expression of thought.

Modern naturopaths tend to place emphasis on the emotional/structural axis with a more *gestalt* approach relating thoughts to feelings and endeavouring to resolve the undischarged impulses, such as anger and grief. The biochemical/emotional axis is also becoming more significant as much of the newer nutritional knowledge establishes clear links between food (as well as other environmental factors) and mental health.

The search for insight into the aberrant emotional compensations is a joint effort of both practitioner and patient which demands a level of intellectual understanding not available in all forms of mental illness. Naturopathic psychotherapy is unsuitable for the treatment of psychotic illness such as the manic-depressive psychoses, or schizophrenia. Nevertheless, naturopaths, with their specialized knowledge of nutrition, may in the future make a significant contribution to the management of such disorders. There is a rapidly accumulating body of evidence to show that individual food sensitivities, as well as deficiencies, may play a role in the causes of mental illness.

We shall consider some of these approaches to mento-emotional disorders which are utilized by naturopaths either directly or indirectly.

Relaxation and Meditation Techniques

As more has been discovered about the physiological mechanisms by which the brain exerts its effects on the body so our understanding of the feedback of information from the body to the brain has increased, and a greater precision in the traditional methods of relaxation used by naturopaths has become possible.

Animal physiology is well attuned to stress, which may be any environmental insult, whether climatic change or physical assault, and not just anxiety or worry. The stress response is a survival mechanism which has enabled each species to evolve and withstand changes in its environment. This is made possible by the adaptation mechanisms described by Selye.[5] In man the evolution of an intellect has enabled him to superimpose certain restraints on the full fruition of these metabolic processes, or to overrule them in a way which can lead to secondary physical tensions. These tensions, which may take the form of muscle spasms, altered breathing rhythms, or other physical symptoms, create affective blocks (obstacles to full expression of thoughts and feelings). Relaxation techniques are designed to reduce these physical tensions and muscle spasms so enabling the patient to give free expression to repressed emotions.

One such approach which has been used by naturopaths for many years is that of L. E. Eeman, in which patients are encouraged to develop an awareness of areas of physical tension in the body and consciously direct a relaxation to them in conjunction with the breathing. 'Sigh, sink, and sag' is an alliteration commonly used to reinforce the imagery. The patient works through the whole body with guidance until he develops sufficient self-awareness to be able to lie down on a comfortable surface and release almost all muscular tension.[6] The Eeman Technique is fundamentally similar to autogenic training which has become popular in recent years.

The principle of conscious self-awareness is also the basis of the biofeedback techniques, in which an electrical skin-resistance meter is used to indicate the degree of arousal or relaxation. As the patient releases tension the instrument provides an audible or visual indication of increased skin resistance which is evidence of a reduction in muscle tone. When practising relaxation the individual endeavours to reduce the intensity of the signal which, therefore, monitors the ability to 'let go'. There is a lowered skin resistance when the body is in a state of arousal or panic.[7]

Another valuable system which reduces physical tensions and promotes a calmer integration of body and mind is the Alexander Technique, referred to in Chapter 6. It is, however, a rather prolonged system of training necessitating a regular commitment for many months but this may be said of many systems of personal development. Reduction of postural stress by the application of basic Alexander principles can be valuable in minimizing tension.

Human Potential

In recent years there has been a great increase in techniques of psychotherapy and personal growth, created perhaps by the multiple pressures of mid-twentieth century life. These therapies claim to be holistically orientated and, apart from providing comfort and reassurance to the emotionally disturbed, they have afforded a means for the healthy individual to become free of the restraints imposed by early conditioning and irrelevant moral codes. Individuals who have experience in such techniques say that they have a greater capacity to enjoy life and appreciate all that it offers — a fuller realization of human potential. This concept of maximizing the capacity for optimal function has, in the past, been more evident, naturopathically, in relation to physical health than the emotional and spiritual levels, but the totality of man's experience in his environment has always been regarded as of the utmost importance.

The various methods of breaking down physical and emotional obstacles to full personal expression include such practises as dynamic meditation, a series of rhythmic exercises with forced breathing which is said to induce higher levels of consciousness — a phenomenon which may be attributed to the physiological increase of adrenalin, mediated via the sympathetic nervous system. These methods are often used in groups known as encounter groups, and, while many people have developed greater awareness through them, there has been an element of exploitation and cultism. Some intensive 'instant enlightenment' courses may also be a danger to individuals whose defensive traits are broken down to expose potentially psychotic tendencies, or when the release is not backed up by sufficient constructive psychological support over a period of time. The more valuable methods of personal growth involve a greater commitment to time, allowing a gradual development of self-awareness with the guidance and support of a skilled therapist.

Among the newer humanistic psychotherapies *Psychosynthesis* recognizes the drive of living matter towards improvement. The purposive vitality (*ponos* of Hippocrates) here becomes conscious as an urge to harmonize and synthesize mental functions at a higher level. While Freudian psychoanalysis was concerned with the recognition of our baser drives, as contained within the subconscious mind, the founder of psychosynthesis, Roberto Assagioli, maintained that there is also a 'super-conscious' which is the origin of the highly evolved impulses of spiritual and philosophical insight. Just as we can suffer from a suppression of our basic biological drives, psychosynthesis suggests, so can we be crippled by 'suppression of the sublime' — a failure to develop our higher nature.[8] Various techniques of meditation, self-analysis, and guided imagery are used to move towards this elevated insight.

Similar techniques are a common feature of *Gestalt psychology* whose basic principle of wholeness comes closest to the unifying approach of naturopathy. The German term *gestalt* means form or structure and its psychology arose in the early decades of the twentieth century as a reaction against the highly analytical views of the time. Gestalt avoids analysis and interpretation and rather addresses itself to the 'positive aspects of personality and living'.[9] The individual's conflicts are seen in terms of his present experience and feelings and the techniques employed encourage the physical and verbal expression of unresolved or suppressed emotions under the sympathetic but non-intrusive guidance of the therapist.

Bioenergetics is again closely related to the naturopathic concepts of structure and function. It derives from the somatic aspect of Wilhelm Reich's theories on energy. He maintained that undischarged bioenergy is bound in the body by the muscles leading to a 'character armouring' which blocks perception and true expression of feelings.[10]

The development of the bioenergetic approach, which involves breathing, body postures, and exercises to develop awareness of tensions, has been largely the work of Alexander Lowen whose methods can be summarized as:

1. Grounding — the discovery of ones own sense of identity.
2. Breathing — the study of breathing patterns. Emotional charge may be increased by physical effort, e.g. kicking or hitting a mattress.
3. Understanding of predominant personality type — Reich described various character structures based partly on the postural attitudes assumed as a reaction to emotional experience.[11]

Physical expression of suppressed emotions also features strongly in many other psychodynamic approaches. *Biodynamic psychology* extends Reich's concept of character armouring to visceral and tissue armouring. The peristaltic waves of the intestines are considered to occur in response to pressures associated with emotional stress.[12] Medicine now recognizes the relationship between the emotions and disorders of the intestinal motility, which may often be labelled an 'irritable colon'.

Primal therapy originates from many sources and relates to the so-called experiences of early childhood which are considered to be the first stages in the production of neuroses. It is considered to be effective where the major psychological conflict involves experiences which occurred before the patient learned to talk, that is from the time of conception to the age of one.

There are other psychotherapeutic approaches too numerous to mention, but which are complementary to the naturopathic holistic approach. Many of these, however, place strong emphasis on the emotional-structural axis of the naturopathic triad. A large number of practitioners place equal, if not more emphasis on the biochemical-emotional axis.

Nutrition and the Mind

Modern research suggests an increasingly strong link between nutrition and the emotional state of the patient. A complex chain of metabolic processes is involved in the conversion of food to energy for the brain and nervous system. When energy is produced an optimum amount of nutrients are required at each stage of the process. If there is a shortage or imbalance of any element at a particular point of the cycle the amount of available energy for the next stage will be insufficient and this, in turn, may be incomplete. Insidiously a state of chronic undernutrition can develop which may lead to psychochemical reactions — alienation from others, distrust, suspicion, and other behavioural traits which may be attributed to biochemical imbalances.

Emotional withdrawal and inability to cope has been observed by Dr George Watson in patients in whom both blood-sugar levels and total fat in the blood were low. According to Watson 80 per cent of the energy produced in the cells is derived from acetate (acetyl coenzyme A) which is an intermediate substance in the transformation of energy from glucose and other substances in the food. Most foods are transformed into acetate by the action of enzymes. Fat is a main source of acetate. Many slimming diets reduce the fat and carbohydrate intake, emphasizing a relatively higher protein content, and the lack of acetate in these diets prevents adequate generation of energy.[13]

One of the major objections to the theory of the physiological basis for mental illness has been the lack of consistency in metabolic findings. Watson suggests that identical symptom complexes can accompany entirely different biochemical anomalies and, conversely, a wide diversity of emotional states may be exhibited by people with essentially similar metabolic disturbances.

Behaviour

Just how far-reaching the effects of an unbalanced diet can be is revealed by studies which have been carried out at various detention centres in the USA. These suggest that a low blood-sugar level can contribute to criminal behaviour.[14]

A chronic low blood-sugar, which may be induced by a diet high in refined carbohydrates and stimulants, such as caffeine in coffee and cola beverages, results in a shortage of energy for brain function leading to irritability, depression, withdrawal, or aggressive tendencies. The mechanism of nutritionally induced hypoglycaemia has been discussed on page 85. The main thrust of the Feingold Diet, which has been found effective in the management of hyperactive children, has been the exclusion of refined carbohydrates and food additives, such as colouring agents or preservatives, which are usually the chemical substances to which the brain cells are sensitive.[14]

Food additives and other environmental toxins, such as lead, are believed to interfere with the functions of some enzymes which play important roles in the metabolic chain of energy production. They may also penetrate the blood-brain barrier to impair the functional ability of the brain cells themselves. Lead is a common environmental poison in industrialized areas, particularly large cities, where traffic fumes may contribute to the high levels from the lead in petrol. Symptoms of toxicity include emotional instability, confusion, depression, and, in young children, mental retardation and hyperactivity.

In 1976 the National Institute of Environmental Health Sciences sponsored a study of Philadelphia children who had no lead poisoning. They found that children with the lowest lead levels had average IQs of 97 whilst those with the highest levels had an average of only 80.[16]

Many food additives have been implicated as a cause of psychotic disorders. A West German study has found that phosphate, commonly used to emulsify products in the food industry, and phosphoric acid, used as a flavour in soft drinks and soft cheese, can alter the behaviour of children. At the University Clinic of Mainz a double-blind controlled study of hyperkinetic and behaviourally disordered children was carried out which indicated that a phosphate-free diet improved the behaviour and learning performance of some of the children.[17] Research increasingly confirms the long-standing naturopathic view that our diet should be free of additives and artificial fertilizers.

Many of these adverse responses to food additives are pharmacological but clinical ecology studies suggest that a number of commonly consumed foods can give rise to allergic reactions with emotional manifestations.

Food Allergy

In Chapter 5 the role of food allergy as a cause of disease was considered. A common feature of such adverse responses to specific foods is emotional disturbance of one form or another and there are many reports of marked behavioural problems being improved by excluding a number of commonly eaten foods from the diet.[18]

A double-blind crossover trial, in which thirty adults were tested with twelve allergens and six placebos, neither patients nor physicians knowing which foods they were given, was reported in 1978. Those exposed to allergens reported a significantly higher incidence of nervous system complaints, including depression, inability to concentrate, anger, irritability, and headaches.[19]

The foods most commonly implicated in these reports are cow's milk, chocolate, cola beverages, eggs, and wheat. Reactions to such everyday items of fare is known as masked food allergy, in which symptoms may occur on withdrawal of the food, or with its re-introduction after a fast or exclusion from the diet for a sufficient time to allow some adjustment. As with many other stressors the body subdues its initial alarm reaction to a stage of resistance while the food is taken regularly but eventually tolerance fails and symptoms return.

Although there is a great deal of corroborative evidence for the naturopathic contention that body chemistry has a profound influence on emotional stability, and a wholefood diet may be at least part of the solution to mental illness, there is clearly need for a great deal more research into this aspect of health. Nevertheless, it might be tempting to suppose that all psychological problems will be found to have a physiochemical basis, and, as food and nutrition are controllable factors, they naturally appeal to the analytically minded for whom a well-defined cause and effect create greater security. In spite of great contributions to the understanding of human behaviour by the psychoanalytic schools, many widely accepted methods of psychotherapy have yet to be proved by scientific methodology. But in an age of the revival of man's intuitive faculties it would be premature to discount the many intangible forces which are part of his being. Certainly few naturopaths would allow themselves to be drawn into an excessively analytical view of the human psyche, if for no other reason than their experience of the subtle power of such adjuncts as plant essences in the management of emotional states.

Prescribing for the Mind

Prescribing by naturopaths for emotional disorders may take the form of supportive nutritional supplements (such as the B vitamins), herbal nervines (nerve sedatives and nutrients), and the Bach Flower Remedies. The latter are a range of plants in potentized form which were discovered in the nineteen twenties and thirties by a physician, Dr Edward Bach. Bach maintained that in medicine one should treat the patient's personality and not his disease. He listed twelve states of mind:

1. Fear.
2. Terror.
3. Mental torture or worry.
4. Indecision.
5. Indifference or boredom.
6. Doubt or discouragement.
7. Over concern.
8. Weakness.
9. Self-distrust.
10. Impatience.
11. Over-enthusiasm.
12. Pride and aloofness.

Bach eventually discovered a range of 38 remedies which could be of benefit to patients suffering from these states of mind.

Mimulus *(Mimulus guttatus)*, for example, is said to help overcome fear from known reasons — such as fear of cancer, fear of flying, or stage fright — by inducing the qualities of 'quiet courage to face trials and difficulties with equanimity'. More extreme terror and apprehension for no known reason is an indication for Aspen *(Populus tremula)*, according to the Bach system of prescribing.[20]

The plants are prepared by placing them in dishes of fresh water in the sunlight at the site of collection. This extracts the therapeutic 'frequency' of the plant in a principle something akin to that of homoeopathic potentization. Some species are potentized by a boiling method. From these stock preparations the patient's prescription, consisting of one or more ingredients, is prepared and minute quantities are administered in liquid several times daily or, perhaps, more frequently in an emergency such as shock.[21]

No biochemical or physiological explanation of the effects of these remedies is evident at present. We may surmise some common vibrational frequency between the plant and the patient's state of mind.

The Bach Flower Remedies are totally compatible with naturopathic principles in catering for the individuality of the patient while also acting as a catalyst to self-healing processes. They may not always remove the need for psychotherapeutic exploration of the roots of the patient's anxiety, impatience, distrust, or whatever, but they can provide preliminary, and sometimes adequate support to enable him to regain sufficient emotional equilibrium.

The Mind as Healer

One aspect of human potential which naturopaths always try to develop is the capacity of the mind to create an environment conducive to healing within the body. There has been more objective investigation of this phenomenon in recent years, for example the work of Dr Carl Simonton on visualization in cancer, and other diseases, is receiving more attention and he has vindicated Henry Lindlahr's view that '. . . affirmations of health are justifiable in the face of disease. Health conditions must first be established in the mind before they can be conveyed to or impressed upon the cells'.[22]

Simonton's method involves training patients to visualize the healing mechanisms of the body at work and he claims success in arresting the progress of many types of cancer.[23]

Conclusion

The vicissitudes and potential of the human mind are still largely uncharted and cannot be encompassed by one set of theories or therapeutic techniques. Within its vitalistic framework, naturopathy has the flexibility of approach to explore the many facets of the psyche and, with newer discoveries corroborating its holistic views, it may make a more positive contribution to the development of human potential in the future.

REFERENCES

[1] Hazzard, A. J., 'Brief Psychotherapeutic Sessions in General Practice', *Practitioner* 227, January 1983, p.107-109.

[2] Lindlahr, H., *Philosophy of Natural Therapeutics* (Revised Edition), Maidstone Osteopathic Clinic, 1975.

[3] Alexander, F., *Psychosomatic Medicine*, Allen & Unwin, London, 1952.

[4] Powell, M., *An Outline of Naturopathic Psychotherapy*, British College of Naturopathy and Osteopathy, London, 1967.

[5] Selye, H., *Stress of Life*, McGraw Hill, Toronto, 1976.

[6] Eeman, L. E., *Co-operative Healing*, Frederick Müller, London, 1947.

[7] Blundell, G., Biofeedback, *Visual Encyclopaedia of Unconventional Medicine*, Trewin Copplestone Publishers Limited, London, 1979.

[8] Assagioli, R., *Psychosynthesis: A Manual of Principles and Techniques*, Viking Press, London, 1971.

[9] Fausset, U., Gestalt Psychology, *Visual Encyclopaedia of Unconventional Medicine, ibid.*

[10] Reich, W., *Character Analysis*, Vision Press, London, 1950.

[11] Lowen, A., *Physical Dynamics of Character Structure*, Grune and Stratton Inc., New York, 1958.

[12] Boyeson, G. and Boyeson, M.-L., Psycho-peristalsis, *Energy & Character*, Vols. 5:1 to 7:3, Abbotsbury, Dorset, 1974-1976.

[13] Watson, G., *Nutrition and Your Mind*, Harper and Row, New York, 1972.

[14] Schauss, A., *Diet, Crime, and Delinquency,* Parker House, Berkeley, California, 1980.
[15] Feingold, B., *Why Your Child is Hyperactive,* Random House, New York, 1975.
[16] Fogel, M. L., 'Auto-fumes may Lower your Kids I.Q.', *Psychology Today,* 13(8):108, January, 1980, quoted in Schauss, A. *ibid.*
[17] Schauss, A., *ibid,* p.59.
[18] Mackarness, R., *Not All In The Mind,* Pan Books, London, 1976.
[19] King, D. S. and Mandell, M., 'A double blind study of allergic cerebro-viscero-somatic malfunctions evoked by provocative sub-lingual challenges with allergen extracts'. *Proc. 12th Advanced Seminar in Clinical Ecology,* Key Biscayne, Florida, 1978.
[20] Hyne-Jones, T. W., *Dictionary of Bach Flower Remedies,* Banstead, Surrey, 1977.
[21] Weeks, N., *The Medical Discoveries of Edward Bach, Physician.* C. W. Daniel, Saffron Walden, 1973.
[22] Lindlahr, H., *ibid,* p.284.
[23] Simonton, O. C., Simonton, S. M. and Creighton, J. L., *Getting Well Again,* Bantam Books, New York, 1980.

9. Naturopathic Medicine in Practice

The general title of this series might imply that naturopathy, and the other natural therapies, are able to provide a complete medical service which can replace conventional medicine. Although it is concerned with the very basics of health care, being, in essence, the art of healing which modern medicine has lost in its rush towards technology and pharmacology, naturopathy is not completely self-sufficient and could not replace the emergency services and life-saving procedures of orthodox medicine. The tremendous scale on which the latter has to operate may sometimes make it seem dehumanizing and impersonal but its analytical approach has created a system which can, in some circumstances, take over where the *vis medicatrix naturae* leaves off.

Accidents or severe infections, where the body's vital reserve is overwhelmed, demand radical measures in the form of surgery or even drugs in the short term. In chronic illness where obstacles to proper function are clearly beyond the control of the body's homoeostatic mechanisms, surgical intervention may remove the impediment and allow self-healing processes to continue more effectively.

The precepts on which naturopathy is based are an essential foundation to other forms of medical care and its techniques play an important role in potentiating the healing process. Although fundamental differences of outlook have to be recognized there is no doubt that naturopathy and conventional medicine will enjoy an increasingly reciprocal relationship in the future. This is already evident in the growth of mutual respect and co-operation between the professions in recent years. Many doctors now refer their patients to naturopaths and osteopaths and willingly exchange the results of tests and investigations which have been carried out in the National Health Service.

This co-operation need not undermine the autonomy of the professions. The two systems are in many ways complementary but, because of their different philosophies and therapeutic emphases, they are undoubtedly alternative modes of medical care. The choice must remain with the patient although the suitability of one or the other approach should be determined by his condition and constitution, a decision which may have to be made with professional guidance. In an era of closer liaison between doctors and the naturopathic profession it may be possible to decide which form of treatment is most appropriate for the individual patient at a particular point in time. As the patient's condition changes so may the treatment required need a new direction.

Only by pooling the resources, skills, and educational capabilities of all sides of the caring professions can we build a true science of medicine which may relieve the presently over-burdened health services.

The Scope of Naturopathy

The word 'doctor' means teacher, and, although they may not use the designation, unless, of course, they hold a medical degree, naturopaths consider one of their most important roles to be educators in health. Their principle task is to determine their patients' potential for health and show them how they may realize it.

There is also a great deal of fear about illness which has been bred of the belief that it is largely the result of external circumstances over which we have no control. A naturopath endeavours to place responsibility for health fairly and squarely back in the hands of the patients by enabling them to understand what the body is trying to do when it is unwell.

In terms of its efficacy, naturopathy is clearly most successful in the functional disorders, those conditions in which pathological changes have not yet taken place in the organs or tissues.

Naturopaths emphasize that they treat patients and not diseases, so avoid labelling symptoms and syndromes with a diagnosis which they consider anyway to be meaningless in terms of the patient's capacity to recover. In considering a skin rash, for example, its precise nature is far less important than the integrity of the patient's gastro-intestinal and respiratory systems.

Nevertheless, it is convenient to classify diseases according to the systems in which their symptoms are manifest and the following are some of the problems with which naturopaths are commonly presented:

Respiratory disorders	— colds, coughs, catarrh, sinusitis, tonsillitis and glandular disturbances, ear problems, bronchitis, asthma, emphysema.
Skin disorders	— dermatitis, eczema, psoriasis, acne, urticaria, boils, and miscellaneous rashes.
Allergic disorders	— which may affect any part of the body but commonly the skin, respiratory system, and digestive system.
Gastro-intestinal disorders	— indigestion, peptic ulcers, gall-bladder and liver diseases, pancreatic disturbances, diarrhoea, constipation, diverticulitis, diverticulosis, colitis.
Cardio-vascular disorders	— high blood-pressure, low blood-pressure, heart weakness and irregularities, atherosclerosis, venous stasis (varicose veins and haemorrhoids), oedema.
Haematological disorders	— disturbances of the blood, such as anaemia.
Genito-urinary disorders	— diseases of kidneys, bladder, and prostate, such as cystitis, urethritis, incontinence, and prostatitis.

Gynaecology	— menstrual and menopausal disorders, pre-menstrual syndrome, prolapse and uterine displacements.
Neurological	— headaches, migraine, neuralgia.
Musculo-skeletal	— back and joint injuries, strains and sprains, rheumatism and arthritis.
Mento-emotional	— tension and anxiety states, irritability, depression, phobias, insomnia.

Naturopathy is used successfully in all these conditions but in many of them there can be disorders of varying acuity and gravity which require conventional medical treatment. Among the musculo-skeletal disorders most injuries can be successfully treated naturopathically but bone fractures are clearly in need of the special skills available in a hospital orthopaedic department. In other systems of the body much may depend on the pathology and general health of the patient. A fibroid of the uterus, for example, may well be contained healthily, or even reduced, by naturopathic treatment, but if it is too large to respond, or causes pressure on other structures such as the bladder, then surgical removal may be the best course of action. This is clearly a case for closer co-operation between doctor, surgeon, and naturopath to guide the patient and fulfil her wishes.

The readiness of the naturopath to treat such emergencies as bronchial pneumonia or meningitis will depend on his familiarity with the patient's health history. Some naturopaths claim to have treated these conditions successfully by a combination of fasting and hydrotherapy, but most practitioners would only treat patients who had been under naturopathic care previously and whose constitution would be capable of the necessary vital response. In the frail or elderly the natural course of the illness may be to overwhelm the body defences and, in such circumstances, conventional antibiotic treatment might be the appropriate life-saving measure.

The health constructive principles of naturopathy can play a valuable role in the convalescence of the patient from serious illnesses. Every case has to be assessed on its own merit and this again emphasizes the need for closer liaison between the various medical disciplines.

Other Surgical Emergencies

While life-threatening situations arise which may call for prompt surgical intervention naturopaths maintain that there are many cases in which surgery might be avoided if proper attention to dietary habits and life-style were introduced at an earlier stage. Surgical removal of the gall-bladder is commonly carried out in cases where gall-stones have been detected, yet these may often be effectively eliminated by naturopathic procedures and prevented by a diet high in fibre and low in refined carbohydrates and animal fats. Candidates for spinal surgery are frequently saved from this by the combination of naturopathic and osteopathic procedures which can restore adaptation to a chronically weak back.

Naturopaths are in agreement with other medical experts who suggest that some organs are removed unnecessarily, since the real cause of the illness lies elsewhere. Enlarged tonsils, often removed in the past, are simply a symptom of a more general lymphatic crisis and catarrhal problem which can, in most circumstances, be treated naturopathically.

Care of the Young

Naturopathic care is particularly suitable for children. The young metabolism is more rapid and vigorous, and many more acute and self-limiting diseases occur. Most of the childhood ailments, such as measles, mumps, and chicken pox, help to confer better immunity for the future and, with proper nursing, the child who is normally well nourished appears to be less susceptible to the complications of these diseases.

Fasting, hydrotherapy, and other forms of eliminative control are effective ways of treating the acute fevers, and gradual constitutional treatment with dietetic guidance is of benefit in many of the more persistent ailments such as asthma, eczema, tonsillar, and other catarrhal problems which so frequently beset children.

An understanding of the nature of disease (see Chapter 2) can remove much of the anxiety parents may feel about the sometimes violent nature of the child's illness. Antibiotics are seldom, if ever, necessary, since, with naturopathic guidance, the body's self-regulatory mechanisms are capable of dealing effectively with most crises. Clinical experience suggests that the proper natural resolution of coughs, colds, and influenza, without suppressive treatment, reduces the likelihood of bronchitis, arthritis, and other degenerative disorders in later life, though long-term research would be needed to establish the validity of this observation with more certainty.

Care of the Elderly

Naturopathic medicine also has an important contribution to make in geriatric care. There may often be limitations to the recuperative response in the older individual but there is scope for various anabolic measures with therapy geared to the vital reserve of the patient.

The nutritional status of the elderly is one area which is badly neglected even in the industrialized nations. A study carried out in the USA showed that among the elderly, 50 per cent suffer from various degrees of deficiency.[1] Another study of subjects ranging in age from 60 to 95 revealed deficiencies in the levels of vitamins B_2 and B_6. Among institutionalized individuals 34.2 per cent were deficient in vitamin B_2 and 56.6 per cent in vitamin B_6, while of subjects in private homes the figures were 27.7 per cent and 42.5 per cent respectively.[2]

Musculo-skeletal problems in the elderly are less amenable to manipulative procedures but the neuro-muscular technique, applied by naturopaths, provides a gentle way of giving relief from these disorders.

At the psychological level the elderly may experience negative emotions associated with a sense of physical decline and naturopaths try to inculcate an attitude that encourages the constructive use of existing resources coupled with the bonus of wisdom and experience which comes with advancing years.

Preventive Medicine

Prevention is something close to the heart of every naturopath. The early detection of abnormalities is of great value to enable practitioners to initiate appropriate treatment, but may, in the view of many naturopaths, detract from the importance of health education.

'We need to interest individuals, communities, and society as a whole in the idea that prevention is better than cure', wrote the authors of *Prevention and Health: Everybody's Business* in 1976,[3] implying that individual responsibility for the basic essentials of living must not be abrogated to high technology, great though its benefits may be.

It is clear that, because of its holistic health-promoting orientation, naturopathy is a preventive system *par excellence.* Preventive medicine has become associated with hygienic measures, vaccination, and mass screening which are inclined to remove the element of personal responsibility for health. Naturopaths have long believed that such measures may encourage the neglect of the real causes of disease and that the resources applied to sophisticated investigations may, in some cases, be better used for education into the importance of better nutrition and life-style as preventives of illness.

The value of screening programmes is debated even in medical circles, where some authorities have drawn attention to the slight risks attached to invasive investigations, such as mammography (X-ray investigations of the breasts for tumours), which may slightly increase the likelihood of carcinoma.[4] Biochemical profiles may also present an excess of irrelevant data showing mild abnormalities which could merely reflect transient changes in the body's normal metabolism. Such detailed investigations can encourage a preoccupation with minor pathological changes with which the healthy body frequently copes without the individual becoming aware of any symptoms.

Concern is sometimes expressed that people undergoing naturopathic treatment may run the risk of serious disorders going undiagnozed and thereby delay essential medical treatment. Since naturopaths are trained in pathology and physical diagnosis the likelihood of this is no greater than it might be in general practice. There may be cases in which early pathologies are reversed by the self-recuperative power of the body under naturopathic, or indeed, any other treatment before they become evident and only comparative screening programmes could confirm this.

The naturopathic diagnostic approach, which assesses constitution, vital reserve, and nutritional and structural integrity, forms a realistic foundation for preventive health measures. Naturopaths believe, furthermore, that prevention should start with present generations for the sake of the future ones.

Preconceptual care has long been a speciality of naturopaths. Many health conscious couples consult practitioners for general health checks by the assessment of their structural integrity, osteopathically, and their nutritional status, with such investigations as iridology and hair analysis. These assessments are done before conception and, ideally, the introduction of wholefood nutritional programmes should be made two or more years before conception is contemplated, particularly if the nutrient level of the female may have been compromised by the use of the contraceptive pill. The pill has been shown to reduce the levels of both zinc and vitamin C in a significant proportion of cases.[5]

During pregnancy programmes of applied nutrition may need to be continued together with the other preparatory exercise and relaxation routines.

Controversial Issues

Some widely promoted and practised preventive health measures are not accepted unquestioningly in the naturopathic profession. *Vaccination* for the prevention or treatment of disease is not generally advocated by naturopaths. While there may be a short-term protection for individuals at high risk from contagion, the principle of vaccination, according to the naturopathic unitary view of disease, evades the primary factors responsible, which are usually environmental and nutritional. It is argued that the statistical evidence for the efficacy of vaccination in protecting against contagious diseases is unreliable. Careful study of the epidemiology reveals that in many cases the disease was already declining in incidence before the vaccination was introduced. The number of deaths in England and Wales from poliomyelitis, for example, declined by 82 per cent between 1950 and 1956, when there was no vaccination programme, compared with a reduction of 67 per cent in the six years after the introduction of vaccines.[6]

The specific preventive effects of vaccination are also called into question by the evidence that many vaccinated individuals still become victims of the disease against which they are supposedly protected. According to a report by the Poliomyelitis Surveillance Unit, of the 210 deaths from poliomyelitis in the USA in 1960, 77 were fully vaccinated.[7]

Although the deaths, and even the complications of vaccination represent an insignificant proportion of those vaccinated, most naturopaths do not subscribe to the view that these are a small price to pay for the large scale social benefit and protection afforded. While concern has centred around the more immediate hazards, such as brain damage following pertussis (whooping cough) vaccine, there may be long-term consequences in terms of neurological or liver damage which only retrospective studies will bring to light. In the meantime the naturopathic view is that such procedures are better avoided where safe alternatives, such as homoeopathy, are available.

The *fluoridation* of public water supplies is an issue on which naturopathic opinion is divided. The addition of sodium fluoride to the water is believed to be an effective way of giving protection against dental caries. It is based on the observation that the incidence of tooth decay is less among children living in areas where the water naturally contains higher concentrations of calcium fluoride. The fluoride ions are taken up and incorporated in the enamel of the teeth only during the period of growth in childhood.

It is argued that, in the face of the tremendous consumption by children of sugar, sweets, and soft drinks, which are among the principle causes of tooth decay, the addition of fluoride to water can at least afford some protection. The majority of naturopaths object to a treatment which tends to give a false sense of security whilst condoning the use of the causative agents, which may, in any case, disturb health in other ways. They maintain that a change in eating habits must be encouraged in the long run if tooth decay is to be effectively prevented.

A further objection to fluoridation is that the form of fluoride added to water is different from that which occurs in areas of naturally high fluoride content. Sodium fluoride, which would be added to water, is a much less stable compound than naturally occurring calcium fluoride. Sodium fluoride is a cumulative poison which is a powerful enzyme inhibitor and antagonist to various minerals such as iodine, essential for thyroid function. The uptake of sodium fluoride by biological systems is more rapid but also shows great individual variation, so that people with diseases of the kidneys or thyroid gland, for example, may be at greater risk of toxicity. Individual intake and output of water shows such variations that some people may accumulate greater concentrations of the fluoride ions.[8]

Whether or not the proposed concentration of one part per million of sodium fluoride in water supplies is sufficient to prove toxic is still open to debate, but there can be no question that the principle of mass medication, which takes no account of biochemical individuality, is not compatible with naturopathic thought. There is, therefore, a strong ethical objection to the addition of substances, other than those necessary for purification, to public water supplies.

Incurable and Degenerative Diseases

As the acute infectious diseases have been overcome by antibiotics, or controlled by better hygienic conditions, there has been an increase in the incidence of chronic and degenerative disease. This has possibly been compounded by the added burden of toxic residues and chemical wastes from food and the environment which hastens the process of mesotrophy (see Chapter 2).

For many people the diagnosis of an 'incurable disease' or an irreversible pathology, such as degenerative arthritis, instils a great sense of hopelessness which may weaken their determination to take steps to adapt and cope with it. Some may consult a naturopath as a last resort but might be disappointed to find that this offers no greater likelihood of a 'cure' than any other treatment. While the hope of recovery may be limited by many factors, not least an absence of any satisfactory understanding of the nature of the illness, naturopathy can help the patient to overcome the false despair by instilling a constructive attitude to the promotion of the body's adaptive and regulatory processes. The disease may not be reversible but the patient can do much to cope more effectively with it by improving his nutrition and applying hydrotherapy, massage, or relaxation and meditation techniques under the guidance of a practitioner.

Paradoxically, it is in the management of cancer, a disease which generates much fear, and may overwhelm the body defences more than most, that naturopathic measures have gained greatest attention recently. Guidance in the application of a wholefood diet, counselling — often in groups where patients with similar illnesses can share their experiences without the usual taboos about discussing the subject — and instruction in relaxation methods, all appear to help in overcoming the 'victim' mentality, and in releasing the will to live which is such an important ingredient of coping with cancer, or any other 'terminal' disease. Even in those cases who cannot arrest the progress of their disease, the sense of doing something positive to help themselves improves the quality of life and makes death, when it is inevitable, a more tranquil and peaceful event for both the patient and their family and friends.

The objective of cancer help centres is not so much to offer a cure but to create conditions in which the patient can develop his own resources to their fullest potential.

For the patient who has to take drugs, or other destructive forms of treatment, such as radiation, naturopathic applied nutrition may be of value to offset the deficiencies these treatments may create.

Research

One of the most frequent criticisms of naturopathy in the past has been lack of scientific verification. There is, it is true, a dearth of objective documentation on many of the basic naturopathic procedures but there are many difficulties inherent in the currently acceptable research methods as far as their application to natural therapies is concerned.

In medical science the double-blind trial is regarded as a reasonable way of ruling out the element of suggestion when a particular treatment, say a new drug, is being tested. Patients with similar complaints, such as high blood-pressure, are divided into two groups, matched for age, sex, and other variables, and one group receives the active drug, the other a placebo (an imitation of the medicine consisting of some inert substance). In the double-blind method neither the patient nor the physician knows who is receiving the active drug so it is possible to be reasonably sure that any significant improvement in patients taking it is not due to other factors. But the methodology appropriate for the testing of drugs cannot be applied to much of the naturopathic repertory. The patient must play such an active part in their treatment that it is impossible to disguise it. Either they apply compresses or they don't; withold some foods or eat others; have their neck adjusted or not. There is little scope for scientific subterfuge in naturopathic treatment.

There is no doubt that the naturopathic profession has dragged its feet in assessing and recording its techniques. Attempts to evaluate naturopathic procedures in practice have been singularly unsuccessful. When in the late 1960s the Research Society for Natural Therapeutics attempted to survey the range of naturopathic approaches to migraine the response from its members (some of the most progressive and enthusiastic practitioners in the country) was so poor as to render the investigation worthless. Most practitioners are too busy to engage in surveys and complete questionnaires. A further obstacle to research in practice is that naturopaths have an obligation to do all they can to help their patients, particularly as they often come after having been through various medical investigations and would not readily submit themselves to further experimentation. This means that the practitioner cannot withold additional advice or treatment, which he believes to be of benefit, simply to assess whether or not the main therapeutic recommendation is effective.

Furthermore, the vital humanistic ingredient of any naturopathic consultation or treatment cannot easily be isolated from the other benefits to the patient. The fact that he receives time, individual attention, sympathy, and encouragement, may be a potent force in the improvement of the patient's health which makes it difficult to evaluate the true worth of the advice and treatment given by the naturopath. Many naturopaths would, in any case, question whether it really matters if the patient's recovery is due to suggestion or physical phenomena as long as it is lasting.

Little or no research is carried out in the academic establishments as many of the lecturers and instructors at these are practitioners who cannot spare further time to supervise research projects. Naturopathic research does not, of course, attract the sort of commercial sponsorship which is bestowed on medical establishments since the drug companies and most large food manufacturers are unlikely to benefit by the success of naturopathic treatment.

It is clear that a new research methodology needs to be devised for the natural therapies and that investigation needs to be carried out by some independent agency which has access to suitable resources, both financial and scientific, and which can draw on the expertise of qualified naturopathic practitioners as well as members of the medical and scientific community. Fortunately organizations, with representatives from all sides of the medical world, have been established to explore new paradigms of investigation.

There are certainly other ways in which the validity of the therapies can be evaluated which might, for example, involve a co-operative enquiry between scientists, practitioners, and patients. Since patients are encouraged to become more responsible for their own health it seems only logical that they should play an active role in discovering the best way of achieving it.

Status of Naturopathy

The unitary principles of disease and the promotion of self-healing mechanisms by the use of non-invasive techniques of medical care have been largely upheld by those outside the established medical profession, in particular naturopathy, although increasing numbers of doctors are now adopting a more holistic approach, applying some of the principles outlined in this book, and reducing their prescription rate. Naturopathy in most parts of the world has developed independently of the medical profession, establishing its own administrative bodies and training schools. The fundamental difference of philosophy between the unifying vitalistic concepts of naturopathy and the reductionist approach of orthodox medical science has necessitated this dichotomy.

In the United Kingdom there is no statutory legislation governing naturopathy, osteopathy, and other unorthodox therapies, so most naturopaths practise under Common Law, which permits anyone to practise anything for which there is no existing legislative control. The practice of medicine and dentistry, for example, are controlled by government Acts, but it is possible for people to set themselves up as naturopaths, or other therapists, with little or no training. The public have, however, been safeguarded by the establishment of professional associations who uphold standards of practice and ethical conduct to which their members must adhere. They have consistently endeavoured to create and maintain high standards of training through their colleges.

The two oldest established professional bodies of naturopathy in the UK, The British Naturopathic and Osteopathic Association (BNOA), and The Incorporated Society of Registered Naturopaths (ISRN), may be traced to a common origin in the Nature Cure Association over sixty years ago. Members of the BNOA are graduates of the British College of Naturopathy and Osteopathy and may use the designatory letters ND (Naturopathic Diploma), and DO (Diploma in Osteopathy), and are entitled to describe themselves as 'Registered Naturopath and Osteopath'. They may also append their association membership as MBNOA. Members of the ISRN are not allowed to use designatory letters other than those of university degrees which they may possess. They may, however, place the description 'Registered Naturopath', and 'Graduate of the Edinburgh School of Natural Therapeutics' (their training college) after their name.

Members of the BNOA are not permitted to advertise other than a standard format announcement by the association when they are first opening a practice in a new district. The ISRN permit their members to place advertisements in the form of professional cards in recognized health magazines, but neither association allows their members to list conditions treated or therapies used in such announcements or on professional stationery.

Professional Codes of Practice conform with those of the medical doctors in respect of confidentiality, referral to colleagues, treatment of minors, and other ethical considerations. Because of the time which must be given to each patient almost all naturopaths are in private practice and charge fees, which may vary according to the area and the overheads of the practice, but these generally fall within guidelines laid down by the associations.

At the time of writing the major private medical insurance companies do not reimburse the fees for naturopathic or osteopathic treatment. The BNOA has regularly made representations to these organizations, arguing that their member's patients are denied cover for a form of treatment which is not available in conventional medicine, and which is, in any case, considerably less costly than most other private medical care.

Naturopaths may sign Sickness or Incapacity Certificates which the Department of Health and Social Security will accept on the same terms as those from GPs. As far as Death Certificates are concerned, coroners will usually accept only those signed by a registered medical practitioner, but naturopaths do not seem to be unduly concerned by the absence of this facility!

The number of naturopaths practising in the UK is still very small, the combined membership of the BNOA and ISRN being approximately 250. There may be a few hundred practitioners of other disciplines, such as osteopathy and acupuncture, giving some sort of naturopathic advice to their patients. A report on *The Status of Complementary Medicine in the UK* by Stephen Fulder and Robin Munro revealed that many practitioners of other natural therapies give advice on diet and life habits at least once to every patient they see.[8]

Naturopathy Overseas

In European countries the Napoleonic Law, by contrast to the Common Law of the U.K., permits the practice of only those professions for which legislation exists. Many naturopaths, therefore, practice 'illegally', or under cover of a recognized professional qualification, such as physiotherapy.

In Holland an active naturopathic association has received sympathetic attention from the Dutch government, which set up a Commission on Alternative Medicine to look into the question of registration. In France the opposition of the medical profession has created a more hostile environment, but a strong tradition of natural medicine has enabled naturopaths to survive in one form or another.

The profession is strongest in Germany, where *Heilpraktikers* (health practitioners) have registration and parity of status with doctors. The Deutsche Heilpraktikerschaft EV, the major professional association, has several thousand members. In Australia a Committee of Enquiry, reporting in 1977, recommended state registration of various professions of natural therapy but not of naturopathy, which it considererd to be 'unscientific and at the best of marginal efficacy', although it was suggested that controls should be exercised over its practice.[9] The Yellow Pages directories for the major cities list a considerable number of naturopaths, but as in the UK, not all of these belong to established professional associations.[10]

The freedom of practice varies according to State Law in the USA. Certain states, such as Arizona, Washington State, Nevada, and Oregon, have set up State Boards to supervise examination of students who have undergone a four year training course, before awarding a licentiate. A number of other states, however, do not permit the practice of unorthodox therapy by non-medical personnel.[11]

State licensing is also the form of practice control in South Africa where approximately 400 practitioners are supervised by the South African Associated Health Services Professions Board.[12]

A Career in Naturopathy

With the rapidly growing public interest in nutrition, exercise, and other ways of maintaining health, coupled with a concern about many of the conventional ways of treating disease, there is an even greater need for the professional skills and guidance which naturopaths can offer. There are still many towns in the UK which do not have a naturopathic practice and it may, therefore, be a worthwhile and rewarding career. The special training in the philosophy of natural therapeutics, the nature of disease and the management of eliminative control and healing crises which the naturopath receives gives a more complete educational foundation for the practice of natural therapy than is available to many other health professionals who may adopt naturopathic modalities.

The Edinburgh School of Natural Therapeutics and The British College of Naturopathy and Osteopathy (BCNO) in London both offer four-year full time courses leading to qualifying examinations, after which successful graduates may become members of the ISRN or the BNOA respectively. The curriculum of the BCNO includes tuition in the following topics:

First year — anatomy, physiology, philosophy of natural therapeutics, principles of osteopathy, soft-tissue techniques, nutrition.

Second year — physiology, pathology, osteopathy, nutrition, clinical dietetics, hydrotherapy.

Third year — clinical theory and practice, osteopathy, orthopaedics, paediatrics, psychology.

Fourth year — clinical practice, X-ray diagnosis, laboratory diagnosis, osteopathy, gynaecology, pharmacology, medical jurisprudence.

Entry requirements to the BCNO are A levels in biology, physics, and chemistry, and O level in English language. Some counties award grants towards the cost of education.

The Future

As the demand for naturopathy, and other alternative therapies, increases there is a more urgent need for some form of legislation to control the registration of practitioners as a safeguard for the public. At present it is possible for anyone to practice naturopathic modalities without any training in the theoretical and clinical foundations upon which they are based. Many of these people do pay attention to individual requirements and, therefore, claim to be 'holistic', but they are misusing the term, as they frequently neglect the important interactions which regulate human health.

The only way the public can be sure of properly qualified guidance is to consult members of the professional associations mentioned in these books. These associations, for their part, are actively exploring paths to official recognition with the aid of parliamentary and legal experts. They do so not to seek any monopoly over the art of healing, which must remain very much a personal responsibility of the individual, but to consolidate and uphold the standards of training and clinical expertise which they have worked for so long to establish.

Meanwhile, with closer co-operation between doctors, scientists, and natural therapists, new research is confirming and refining many well-tried naturopathic procedures. In the field of nutritional biochemistry, for example, rapid advances are correlating many of the prominent features of naturopathic dietetics and closer links between psychological states and body physiology are being established.

Patients have freedom of choice in medical treatment but can only exercise this when there is a strong naturopathic profession able to provide a comprehensive alternative and not simply palliative measures which may be no better than the drugs they seek to avoid. It is not sufficient for the patient to be relieved of his pain by manipulation, or cold packs, or subjected to some dietary dogma, without being instructed in ways of preventing the disorder in the future. Therapy and education must be matched to the needs of the individual patient.

All systems of medicine are moving towards a more humanistic and complementary role, each having its functions to perform in a given situation, and within this more enlightened era of medical care naturopathy will surely feature most strongly as the guardian of the foundations of health.

REFERENCES

[1] Revlin, R., 'Nutrition and Ageing', reported in *J. of Alternative Medicine*, August 1983.

[2] *International J. Brit. Nutr. Res.* 51, 232-238, 1981.

[3] *Prevention and Health: Everybody's Business*, H.M.S.O., 1976.

[4] Jackson, R., 'Introduction to Symposium on Screening', *The Practitioner*, 225, May 1981, p.623.

[5] Grant, E., 'The Contraceptive Pill: Its Relation to Allergy and Illness', *Nutrition and Health* 2:1, 1983.
Lodge-Rees, E., 'The concept of pre-conceptual care', *Intern. J. Environmental Studies*, 1981, Vol. 17, pp.37-42.

[6] Nightingale, M., 'Poliomyelitis', *Epoch* 5:4, 1983.

[7] *Poliomyelitis Surveillance Unit Report* 224, June 1961, US Department of Health, Education and Welfare, Public Health Service.

[8] Smith, E., 'Fluoridation — are the dangers resolved?', *New Scientist* 5 May 1983, pp. 286-287.

[9] Fulder, S. and Munro, R., *Status of Complementary Medicine in the United Kingdom*, Threshold Foundation, London, 1981.

[10] Report of the Committee of Enquiry into Chiropractic, Osteopathy, and Naturopathy (The Wolff Enquiry), Australia, 1977.

[11] L. Fisher, D.C., personal communication, August 1983.

[12] Gil Alvarado N.D., personal communication, May 1983.

[13] Joyce Harvey BAc, personal communication, September 1983.

Useful Addresses

British Naturopathic and Osteopathic Association
Frazer House
6 Netherhall Gardens
London NW3 5RR

Publishes manifesto and register of qualified practitioners.

Incorporated Society of Registered Naturopaths
1 Albermarle Road
The Mount
York YO2 1EN

Publishes directory of qualified practitioners.

British College of Naturopathy and Osteopathy
Frazer House
6 Netherhall Gardens
London NW3 5RR

Full-time academic and clinical training leading to qualifying examinations.

Society of Teachers of the Alexander Technique
3b Albert Court
Kensington Gore
London SW7

Directory of recognized teachers.

Dr Edward Bach Centre
Mount Vernon
Sotwell
Oxon OX10 0PZ

Books and remedies on the Bach Remedy Repertory.

Human Potential Resources
LFG Ltd.
HP 12
Subscription Department
P.O. Box 10
Lincoln LN5 8XE

Magazine and directory for the human potential movement.

McCarrison Society
23 Stanley Court
Worcester Road
Sutton
Surrey

Studies relationship between health and nutrition.

Research Council for Complementary Medicine
Suite 1
19a Cavendish Square
London W1M 9AD

Promotes research into all forms of natural therapy.

Journal of Alternative Medicine
30 Station Approach
West Byfleet
Surrey KT14 6NF

Monthly journal for practitioners of natural therapy.

Foresight
The Old Vicarage
Witley
Godalming
Surrey GV8 5PN

Society for promotion of preconceptual care.

Index